Women and Health: Cultural and Social Perspectives

Handling the Sick

*The Women of St. Luke's and the
Nature of Nursing, 1892–1937*

Tom Olson and Eileen Walsh

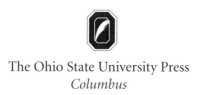

The Ohio State University Press
Columbus

Library of Congress Cataloging-in-Publication Data

Olson, Tom (Tom Craig)
Handling the sick : the women of St. Luke's and the nature of nursing,
1892–1937 / Tom Olson and Eileen Walsh.
p. cm. — (Women and health)
Includes bibliographical references and index.
ISBN 0-8142-0959-9 (hardcover : alk. paper) — ISBN 0-8142-9036-1
(CD-ROM)
1. Nursing—Minnesota—Saint Paul—History. 2. St. Luke's Hospital (Saint Paul,
Minn.)— History. I. Walsh, Eileen. II. Title. III. Women & health (Columbus, Ohio)
RT5.M6 O44 2004
610.73'09776'581—dc22
2003023638

Cover design by Dan O'Dair.
Type set in Minion.
Printed by Thomson-Shore.

9 8 7 6 5 4 3

Contents

List of Illustrations

List of Tables

List of Abbreviations

ANA   American Nurses' Association
MHS   Minnesota Historical Society, St. Paul, Minnesota
MNA/FD   Minnesota Nurses' Association, Fourth District
MNBNE   Minnesota Board of Nurse Examiners
NLNE   National League for Nursing Education
SLHTS   St. Luke's Hospital Training School for Nurses

Preface

Handling the Sick analyzes the rich archival collection of the St. Luke's Hospital and Nurse Training School, documenting the creation, growth, and demise of an early twentieth-century hospital nursing school—a school similar to many others around the country. In it, we hear the voices of applicants, nursing students, rank-and-file nurses, and administrators as we come to understand the motivations that led women into nursing and what the work meant to them, both personally and professionally. The women took pride in their on-the-job training and workplace experience that emphasized the development of their abilities and their character. Tom Olson and Eileen Walsh demonstrate that, for this generation, nursing was not a profession, but a skilled craft. Challenging much of the historiography in the history of nursing, their study is an important contribution to the discipline as well as to women's history and health care history in the twentieth century. We are pleased to publish this provocative study of professional development in the early year's of nursing's formation.

Rima D. Apple
Janet Golden

Acknowledgments

When I made the transition from a history teacher to a nurse, during the mid-1970s, I did so with what I now realize were only hazy notions of what this change would involve. But once tied to the professional aspirations of nursing, by my own ambitions and academic credentials, my first inclination was that my research would help to fan the flame of righteous indignation about nursing's long history of struggle and exploitation. In so doing, I understood that I might help nursing to advance another step further toward the elusive goal of an undisputed, full professional status. After all, most of what I read and heard reinforced the "facts" of nursing's historical trials and tribulations. And so, with a crusader's zeal and a dog-eared copy of Jo Ann Ashley's classic essay on exploitation and early nursing (*Hospitals, Paternalism and the Role of the Nurse* [New York: Teachers College Press, 1976]), I set out to express my allegiance, albeit in scholarly terms, to nursing's professional destiny. Gradually, however, I began to realize the obvious, that what I found might not fit my preconceptions.

I am especially grateful to those individuals who gave me the courage to challenge familiar ways of thinking and to complete this book. My deepest thanks to Bill Lewis, for his steadfast companionship and unfailing patience in reviewing my work; Jeff Stewart, for his generous insights and for always urging me forward; Floris King, for believing in the promise of this undertaking from the beginning; Diane Kjervik, for her wisdom and belief in empowerment; Steve Ruggles, Matt Sobek, and the members of the Social History Research Laboratory for sharing their experience and skill in quantitative analysis; John Eyler, for always listening and inspiring; Debbie Miller and the staff of the Minnesota Historical Society for their enthusiastic support; and Sharon Aadalen, for her foresight in preserving many of the records on which this study is based.

—Tom Olson

The history of working people in the United States deserves careful readings of primary materials such as those provided in the records of St. Luke's. Historians do the best we can with what evidence survives, but we always wish there were more. It was thrilling to see Tom Olson uncover these "new" records that so much improve our understanding of what it meant to be a young working woman in early-twentieth-century Minnesota and in the early field of trained nursing. I am grateful to Tom Olson for inviting me to join him in this project. It bodes well for scholarship when colleagues from different academic fields find they share common intellectual ground and can enhance each other's work.

—Eileen Walsh

We are very grateful for the financial support of the following organizations: Sigma Theta Tau International; the University of Minnesota; Zeta and Gamma Psi Chapters of Sigma Theta Tau International; the American Nurses Foundation (Council on Graduate Education for Administration in Nursing Scholar); the University of Hawaii at Manoa; and the Minnesota Historical Society. Most of all, we are indebted to the women of St. Luke's, both those to whom we were able to speak in person, as well as to those whom we came to know through the records that they left behind. Alternately perplexing, humorous, somber, and inspiring, we could not have asked for better company in this journey of discovery. Nor could we ever thank them enough for their profound teaching about the enduring traditions that lie at the heart of nursing.

1

Introduction:
The Nature of Nursing

It has been said and written scores of times, that every woman
makes a good nurse. I believe, on the contrary, that the very elements of nursing are all but unknown.

—Florence Nightingale[1]

The professionalization framework is the starting point for under
standing the written history of nursing, as this remains the pre-
dominant approach to nursing's past. Two factors help to explain
this. First, professionalization has long been the dominant strategy of nursing leaders. Second, historians of nursing have been inclined to use this
strategy as their framework in interpreting nursing history. Indeed, for
much of nursing's past, the historians and leaders of nursing were one and
the same. As Oderkirk explains, "Nursing history has been counted among
that historiographical species pejoratively called 'in-house' history, written
by practitioners for practitioners, and identified by a propensity toward
hagiography, evangelism, and images of professional destiny."[2]

Underlying this framework is the assumption that nursing is advancing
through a process of professionalization. Among the leaders of nursing, this
idea has been so deeply ingrained that ideas to the contrary are unfath-
omable. Thus, in the texts that are written to help socialize fledgling nurses
into their chosen work, nursing authors regularly exhort their readers to
recall nursing's emergence as a profession from a dark past. Typical of such
treatises, one author remarks, "From its unorganized and poorly defined
beginnings, a profession based on . . . competence, autonomy, determination,
and human caring evolved."[3] Small wonder, then, that doubts about the professionalization of nursing seem almost as improbable as questioning the

nature of nursing itself, which in contemporary discussions is often typified by the phrase "nursing is caring."

Professionalization in nursing is most often viewed as occurring in a series of stages, as professions are typically understood.[4] Progress through each stage is thought to involve certain accomplishments: a focus on academics or theory-driven knowledge, including a constant upgrading of educational standards; consolidation of authority; establishment of state registration and accreditation of schools; and attainment of self-regulation or autonomy. Of course, specific descriptions often vary in terms of the aspect of professionalization emphasized. However, the underlying message remains the same.

Some authors spotlight the consolidation of authority among the major nursing organizations in describing the path to professionalism in nursing. One such individual warns against "the dilution of the profession's strength and the diffusion of its leadership."[5] In a slightly different example, another writer stresses the increased quality and length of nurses' training, along with greater control over their education and work, in tracing "nursing's progress toward professionalism" during the period 1850 to 1920.[6] Another cites "the silent battle" over nurse registration, between 1903 and 1920, as the pivotal factor in the ongoing conflict to distinguish nursing from a skilled trade and to raise it from the status of a "semi-profession" to that of a full profession.[7]

Accounts that boldly raise an alternative explanation of nursing's past tend to quickly revert to familiar patterns. For instance, in an essay entitled "Constructing the Mind of Nursing," a leading nurse historian reflects that "revisionist historical scholars have lately expanded the explanations of nursing's conception beyond 'the great woman theory' of Nightingale's genius'" to encompass a wider array of ideas. Yet venturing only slightly beyond Nightingale, nursing is seen here as a field of "emerging professionals," in an "intellectual terrain" dominated by three of North America's nursing's elite: Lillian Wald, Annie Goodrich, and Lavinia Dock. The outcome is predictable, as the account continues: "And once again, the idea of compassion and caring as a central virtue in nursing appeals to the core of nurses."[8] As this study will explore, caring has become the rallying point for academicians in nursing have sought to define a unique occupational knowledge base that will establish the field's full-fledged professional status.[9]

In a well-researched book on technology, gender, and American nursing, another author similarly promises new insights into the nature of nursing. "Angling for space (with doctors and others) in the 'narrow passageway' leading to the bedside of patients," this individual contends, " . . . nurses believed that the tangibility of things and the visibility of procedures embracing those things would make their knowledge and work more perceptible and discrete." However, incorporating new technologies into nursing practice failed to differentiate this field from other health-related pursuits. As a consequence, nurses eventually "realigned their practice with . . . feminine caring," in an effort "to separate themselves from technology" and to reclaim "'tender loving care' (TLC) . . . as true nursing." This is an interesting interpretation yet, as in the previous example, new information in this narrative for the most part only props up old arguments. Thus, technologizing is described as failing nursing because it did not "fulfill nurses' desires . . . for professional autonomy and visibility." The focus is once again on traditional characteristics of professions and the aspirations of nurses are as tightly bound as ever to the idea of professionalization.[10]

Contrary to the stereotypes suggested by its subjects, a study of nineteenth-century nurses, nuns, and hospitals actually comes the closest of these examples to overturning usual ways of viewing nursing's past. The author sets out to debunk the traditional heroic nursing narrative, focusing instead on the Irish, German, French, and Scandinavian immigrant women who became nursing nuns and deaconesses in North America. She argues that "nursing needs to look beyond the veil and see that its progenitors were not the meek and obedient slaves to medicine that Florence Nightingale and Dorothy Dix would have us believe." With such statements the account challenges traditional approaches to nursing history and bolsters some of the lessons learned from the women of St. Luke's, the focus of our narrative. Still, this study of religion and nursing parallels other descriptions in its ultimate focus, which is the story of how "the sisters overcame the obstacles and restrictions placed in the way . . . as the nursing profession emerged and training became routine." "Pious professionals" are described as presiding over a revolution in "the history of the rise of professional nursing." Thus, rather than offering a significantly different vantage point from which to consider nursing, for the most part Nightingale is simply replaced by another group of heroes who in their turn take up the mantle of professionalization.[11]

These customary ways of viewing nursing all emanate from the assumption that nursing is an emerging profession. Though the works just cited are all from contemporary writers, the basic approach to nursing's past has changed little over time. In an argument that could easily be heard today, a classic history from 1920 emphasizes the need to strengthen the theoretical and scientific side of nurses' training in order to advance the struggle for professional independence and to prevent "the possibility that nursing becomes little more than a trade."[12] The same perspective is echoed twenty-nine years later in Roberts's contention that if apprentice training on the job had not typified early nursing, the evolution of American nursing might have more nearly paralleled that of other professions. More optimistically, Roberts goes on to outline "the triumphs of nursing in its rise . . . toward the stature of a profession."[13] In her praise, she singles out the success of leaders in nursing education, the growth of professional organizations, and the rise of state boards of examiners.

Descriptions such as these, whether from past or present observers, share common threads, including the assumption that the professionalization track accurately portrays nursing history, the implicit belief in the desirability of professionalization as distinct from a trade, and an emphasis on familiar features of professionalization.[14] The predominance of these ideas is perpetuated by incomplete, broad-brush research into the apprenticeship system of work and training that characterized nursing around the turn of the century. Lacking are detailed accounts of apprentice nurses, the key to expanding our understanding of how nursing evolved from the late nineteenth century to the present.

A major work on Nebraska nursing education, for instance, concludes that little direct evidence exists about early training programs because, in general, programs did not keep records. In place of such evidence, the study is typical of others in its dependence on accreditation material from the state board of nursing, along with legislative documents, to infer what apprenticeship in nursing was like. Because these sources recorded the activities of nursing leaders, rather than rank-and-file nurses, the narrative is predictable in reinforcing established notions of professionalization, attributed in this case to "the organizational revolution in nursing."[15]

Documentation from apprentice nurses is also conspicuously absent in a similar investigation of nurses' training in Ohio, covering the years 1892 to 1980. The study focuses on the milestones in the professionalization of nursing, culminating in a lengthy argument in favor of the baccalaureate degree as "the minimum requirement for the professional nurse."[16] Detailed information from students is also missing from a history of Iowa nursing programs, though this does not stop the writer from claiming her study as proof of the "development of a profession."[17] Like the Ohio history, this one also highlights the need to establish minimum educational requirements for nursing.

This consensus in interpretation has made historical conclusions about nursing almost routine, especially in regard to the apprenticeship system of work and training that characterized nursing in the late nineteenth and early twentieth centuries. Thus, Ashley uses her oft-quoted essay to sharply rebuke the apprenticeship system for enforcing "unquestioning subservience."[18] She concludes that it is an unfortunate and repressive part of nursing's past because it impeded nurses' professional development. Picking up this same theme, one of today's most prominent historians of nursing condemns the apprenticeship system for "turning out . . . human machines" and creating a situation "that stymied efforts to achieve professional autonomy."[19] Still others criticize early hospital programs for their "failure to educate for a profession," describing apprenticeship in nursing as "three years of diligent, dreary practice and work" designed to produce "quiet, submissive slave(s)."[20] Or, as a popular contemporary text sums up nursing's apprenticeship past: "school(ing) in submission."[21]

A much less noticed, yet important, alternative to a focus on professionalization concentrates on the craft tradition of nursing. Far from being a form of subservience, early nursing was a skilled field that generated pride in work well done and allowed for relative independence within a context of quite rigid gender roles. This alternative is most clearly presented in the work of Melosh and remains largely unexplored by other researchers. Melosh argues that professionalization offers "a distorting lens for looking at the history of nursing."[22] She explains that historians who adopt this "pervasive paradigm" express the narrow view of a nursing elite, but not the position of the vast majority of nurses. According to the craft-focused framework, the distinctive history of the hospital schools of nursing shaped and strengthened a coherent ideology that offered a powerful option, and even a direct challenge, to the values of professional ideology.[23]

The challenge to professionalization came from nursing's legacy of pride in manual skills, direct involvement with the sick, respect for experience and concomitant mistrust for theory. Academic pursuits were downplayed, while the values of apprenticeship were stressed—empathy and self-discipline rather than intellectual curiosity, carefully honed craft skills rather than research or study. These values led the average nurse to resist the professionalizing efforts of nursing leaders with a defiance that "verged on anti-intellectualism."[24] As one nurse who trained in the 1890s observed, "This underemphasis of the need for skilled craftsmanship . . . seems never to have had import to those nurses who dominate the educational field, and who have clamored so loudly for the recognition of nursing as a profession and not a vocation."[25]

More than half a century later, in the 1960s, another nurse expressed similar sentiments, complaining that an emphasis on academics in nursing was creating a situation in which nurses are "afraid to handle bedpans and give backrubs."[26] During the same decade a hospital staff nurse wrote, "If I am hospitalized, I hope that the nurses who care for me have a thorough education in nursing. I hope that they know pharmacology, aseptic techniques, symptomology, and so on. I shall not care if they know a Van Gogh from a Rembrandt or have six credits in physical education."[27]

As one historian affirms, supporters of apprenticeship education emphasized the importance of craft skills and quality patient care. They proudly defended the virtues of hospital-based education, including "the opportunity to practice techniques and tricky manual procedures until they became second nature, and the chance to work on the wards and benefit from the advice of seasoned veterans."[28]

~

Between these opposing positions lies an occupational divide that has pitted ordinary nurses—the torchbearers of skilled craftsmanship—against nursing leaders—the champions of professional advancement—for more than a century. Nursing literature is replete with references to "the deep divisions within nursing," "the gap that continues to exist between practicing nurses and the American Nurses' Association leadership," and "the huge gulf between what nurses are taught in nursing colleges and the pragmatic . . . approach to nursing that continues to be adopted in many clinical areas."[29] One of the most salient examples of these differences—the controversy involving the necessary preparation to become a nurse—surrounded the opening of the first nursing programs in the United States in the last part of the nineteenth century. The ensuing conflict foreshadowed the present, confusing situation in which basic entry into nursing practice is achieved by any one of three routes: a two-year community college degree, a three-year diploma, or a four-year baccalaureate degree.[30]

With each side continuing to hold "very different beliefs about the nature and purpose (of nursing)," there is little sign of a rapprochement within nursing.[31] Yet there has never been a greater urgency to better understand this impasse. Indeed, we are now faced with a nursing shortage of near catastrophic proportions that shows few signs of diminishing, and there is every indication that internal occupational tensions are as much to blame as external forces for frustrating the aspirations of prospective nurses and prompting many graduates to leave their jobs.[32]

In chronicling the tensions both within and outside of nursing, historians have tended to focus on documenting nursing's progress toward professionhood. Occasionally this has meant seeing nurses struggling against one another, but for the most part it has meant envisioning nurses as moving forward in relative uniformity to overcome shared hardship and adversity. From a craft perspective, though, rank-and-file nurses are more likely to be seen as active participants in an apprenticeship culture rather than victims of a regrettable system of work and training. Of course this assumes that a deeply rooted craft tradition exists within nursing. As luck would have it, evidence of the craft tradition depends on detailed information from those least likely to be represented in the most readily available historical records—average nurses. Most writers, as in the Nebraska example mentioned above, suggest that direct evidence from the rank and file in nursing is nearly impossible to find, leaving us to rely on inferences from scattered fragments and indirectly related sources. Given this situation, it is not so surprising that the record is mostly silent in terms of the developing craft approach to nursing, or of other possible alternatives to professionalization.[33] This is exactly what makes the major source of information for this book, the St. Luke's data, so tremendously valuable.

$\sim$

Despite the passage of time, the voices of the nurses who are at the center of this account are relentless in demanding that we carefully revisit the assumptions that have guided most written histories of nursing. In truth, only a few of the women were available for face-to-face interviews, but their insistence on our seeing their experience for what it was to them, not for what we might want it to be, comes through as well in the rich and detailed material that they left behind. Most of this material has been preserved in the records of the St. Luke's Hospital Training School for Nurses, which operated from 1892 to 1937 in St. Paul, Minnesota.[34] With the unexplained exception of the program's first five years, the collection includes the individual files of all 838 women (graduates and nongraduates) who entered the hospital to become nurses. The files contain letters from the women explaining why they wanted to become nurses; applications that describe their qualifications; reference letters from neighbors, friends, family, and employers; detailed descriptions of their training and education; and records of their experiences after St. Luke's.

Despite the richness of this source, the choice of St. Luke's might seem unusual, given that other studies have tended to focus on exemplary training programs such as those at Johns Hopkins and New York Hospital.[35] But it is exactly the ordinariness of the St. Luke's school, both in historical perspective and as perceived by community groups, accrediting agencies, applicants, nurses, and the public at the time, that make it a particularly useful subject. The school earned a reputation for providing "good training" in a "proper hospital,"[36] admirable traits but not traits unique to St. Luke's. In fact, while the St. Luke's nurses were well respected, none achieved national or even regional prominence. Nor was the school's opening a path-breaking event, or any aspect of its organization and plan particularly stellar. Instead, the program was typical in length, schedule, and focus, simply another part of a nationwide increase in hospital-based training programs. During this era, such programs were the source of nearly all "trained nurses," with the national numbers increasing from 16 in 1880, to 549 in 1900, to more than 1,800 in 1920.[37]

Even in its closing, in 1937, St. Luke's was consistent with national and local trends, in that the number of hospital schools plummeted in the 1930s.[38] The hospital was typical also in terms of its size—150 beds—as well as in its focus on patients with general medical and surgical needs, and in its religious affiliation.[39] Here, then, is an extraordinary collection of information involving an ordinary group of individuals in a standard context. As such, it provides an invaluable window into the historic nature of nursing—the largest healthcare occupation then and now.

Due to the fact that hospitals were dramatically increasing in number and size during the period of study, focusing on a training school to explore the nature of nursing seems especially appropriate. Historians regard "the fusion of the training of nurses with the practice of nursing," as one historian points out, "as the fundamental conflict" of early nursing.[40] Thus, within the apprenticeship system of hospital-based training, more than any other setting, nursing directly confronted issues crucial to its occupational evolution. Here nursing met head-on with the paradigmatic profession of medicine, the emergence of modern science, questions of gender and paid work, and class. These issues frame our research and highlight its broader significance. They also point to the underlying question of this account, "What is the nature of nursing?"

2

First Impressions

I think I should enjoy the work, if one may use such a word in
connection with suffering.

— St. Luke's applicant, 1901[1]

T he women arrived at separate times, throughout 1892, with "two
or three gingham or calico dresses made plainly, six large white
aprons made of bleached cotton with bibs . . . two bags for soiled
clothes, one pair of scissors, a pin ball and a napkin-ring, a good supply of
plain under clothing . . . (and) wear(ing) broad-toed and flat-heeled
boots." As they entered the reception room of the newly opened hospital on
Smith Avenue, the superintendent, Mrs. Bradbury, impressed on each one
that they were privileged to be among the first group of women to enter the
St. Luke's Hospital Training School for Nurses.

They were reminded that "no hospital more perfect in its adaptation to
all the requirements of its work can be found in the land," let alone in St.
Paul. Designed with ventilating shafts and many windows to bring in fresh
air, the building had the latest conveniences, including both gas and elec-
tric lights, speaking tubes, call buttons, and two elevators. Still, the women
were only vaguely aware of the powerful forces surrounding the opening of
the hospital and its training school.[2]

~

The opening of the new St. Luke's (see figure 1), a hospital that traced its
establishment back to 1857, was part of an unparalleled building boom in
its hometown of St. Paul, Minnesota. In the wake of a surge in population
during the 1880s, the number of building permits increased from 729 to
13,102 in just six years. St. Paul was in the midst of a transformation from

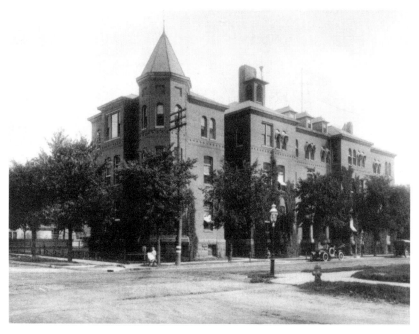

Figure 1. "The New St. Luke's," 1915. From Minnesota Historical Society's Collection #143.B.20.4(B), Box 8, United Hospital Records, Folder: Exterior Views, 1890–1915.

a small, frontier town, characterized by "frame houses and stubby business blocks," to a city of often monumental structures, typifying America's vision of itself during the expansionist era. The city continued to prosper even through the national depression of 1893.[3]

St. Luke's signaled its intent to join the expansionist trend with the discussion of a new hospital at a Board of Trustees meeting in 1883.[4] But the need for a new building went beyond civic competition. The hospital's annual reports from this period indicate that the "old building," which actually was not designed to be a hospital, had outlived its usefulness. It was described as "inadequate in all respects . . . dilapidated . . . (and) falling rapidly into decay."[5] Hospital officials were also interested in attracting additional patients.[6] The annual report for 1889 explained, "This city is filled with young men living in blocks and boarding houses. . . . When sickness comes, remote from parents and friends, the ill results of poor nursing . . . would be theirs were it not for the presence of an institution which provides for them faithful nursing and kindly interest."[7]

The hospital was located in an area where a concentrated number of railroad workers lived, the group to which the report referred. Many were recent arrivals, single men who had responded to an aggressive recruitment effort by prominent Minnesotans and the State Board of Immigration to get workers to build railroads, farmers to till the soil, and tradesmen to supply the farmers. To attract such individuals, the board published pamphlets in German, Swedish, Norwegian, Welsh, and other languages, and sent agents to American seaports and Europe to recruit immigrants. The success of the recruitment effort was born out by census figures that showed, from 1870 to 1920, two-thirds or more of Minnesota's residents were foreign-born or the children of foreign-born parents.[8] Thus, the human setting for St. Luke's included a population that was rapidly expanding, increasingly diverse, and frequently cut off from family support.

In trying to meet the health needs of this changing population, it was no accident that the trustees of St. Luke's specified nursing in their 1889 annual report. That attention to nursing simply reflected the reality of health care near the turn of the century. Scientific medicine was in its infancy during this period and nursing was the primary service that hospitals had to offer. "Until the second quarter of this century," a contemporary professor of medicine observes, "medical treatment had little positive effect on when, or even whether, sick people recovered."[9]

Pointing out the advantages of nursing also made good business sense. Although charity patients were central to the hospital's endeavor to stand as a stronger argument "in favor of Christianity . . . than the church or preachers," it was money that kept the hospital doors open.[10] In the first year of operation at the new St. Luke's 152 patients paid for their care, while endowments and charitable giving paid for the partial or total expenses of only thirty-one patients. Payment for private ward patients was set at $1 per day. Those who could afford a private room paid from $10 to $25 per week. Nonpaying patients were "expected to show a readiness to oblige one another and assist in such services in the wards as their health enables."[11]

Medicine was in a particularly uncertain state at St. Luke's when the first prospective nurses arrived.[12] The twenty-seven physicians who practiced at the hospital in 1892 were in the midst of an intense, nationwide struggle over which school of medicine, allopathy or homeopathy, would take precedence. Practitioners of orthodox medicine had been labeled allopaths, meaning "cure by opposites," by homeopaths and practitioners of other schools of medicine. Those "regular physicians," as they were also described, claimed to be reformers who took the best from various schools and insisted on the importance of empirical knowledge. At St. Luke's, orthodox physicians competed with homeopaths, who were set apart by their belief in the homeopathic "law of similars" ("like cures like") and their use of minute doses of drugs to treat patients.[13]

It is evidence of the tenuous nature of medicine at this time that the two groups regularly disagreed—about what they would be called, the number of physicians from each group that would be allowed at St. Luke's, the wards on which each would practice, and, of course, the success of their treatment approaches.[14] Such competition even spilled over to rivalries between patients. An allopath at the hospital recalled the following contest between two patients over who would recover the fastest: "Side by side in the same ward, the late Dr. Henry Hutchinson and I had a typhoid patient apiece. My patient was getting on better than the other man, and he ragged him, boasting of the superiority of the allopathic treatment. Suddenly he grew much worse while Dr. Hutchinson's patient shot ahead and made a good recovery to the great glory of the homeopathic school and the disgust of my allopathic patient who had laughed too soon."[15]

One thing all the physicians shared was gender: they were men, which generally meant they were foremost in societal power, relative to women. In the absence of a single, dominant physician group, however, the day-to-day affairs of St. Luke's were in the hands of women. Two groups comprised entirely of women—the Board of Managers and the Visiting Committee—were responsible for the conduct of most regular business at the hospital from 1873 until 1901. The Board of Trustees, which was an all-male group, accepted virtually all of the women's suggestions. The rival physician groups, also all male, had no other choice but to acquiesce until years later, as the influence and authority of the orthodox physicians grew and the balance of power eventually tipped toward their rule.

For reasons now unknown, the "lady managers" decided to reorganize the medical staff in 1900. It was their undoing. Their mistake, according to Dr. C. Lyman Greene, the physician appointed chief of staff, was "taking it upon themselves to nominate and elect an entirely new staff without consulting the medical men themselves." The physicians, in total, "declined to have anything to do with a staff elected that way" and proceeded with their own reorganization. Dr. Greene then launched a blistering attack on current management, insisting (less than a decade after the opening of the new hospital) that "the present facilities at St. Luke's are entirely inadequate and not in keeping with the wealth and importance of the city of St. Paul, nor with the magnitude of the work therein attempted." In addition to a new management structure, he declared that St. Luke's should become "the nucleus of a larger non-sectarian hospital," with expanded support "to include certain of our wealthy and influential citizens."[16]

Just six months after the standoff between the lady managers and the physicians, at a special meeting of the trustees, it was agreed to change the composition of the Board of Managers "so as to meet the approval of the

Board of Physicians."[17] The lady managers, who for so long had been directly responsible for guiding hospital affairs, all lost their positions to men, mostly physicians. This shift in power seemed to occur swiftly. Yet as with most things historical it was part of a gradual process, witnessed by a steady increase in the prestige of scientific medicine, the consolidation of power among orthodox physicians, and the resultant decrease in sectarianism among medical practitioners. Although hospital tradition was on their side, the lady managers were no match for a revitalized and more unified group of medical men. In a footnote to their ouster, the St. Luke's Visiting Committee remained the exclusive domain of women. However, this group posed little threat to the new balance of power. Members tacitly agreed to confine their work to "fundraising and sewing."[18]

Victory for the medical staff did not alter the fact that the main offering of the hospital in 1900, just as in 1892, was nursing. The success of the hospital depended heavily on the success of the school, as the majority of nursing work was done by the women who came for training. This was true not only at St. Luke's but across the country.[19] Thus, the first actions of the newly organized Board of Managers, now under the authority of the Board of Physicians, focused on nursing. The managers approved the purchase of another building in order to "furnish better accommodations for the nurses," observing that "the nurses at St. Luke's at present are huddled in ill-ventilated, improperly heated and ill-lighted buildings that are a disgrace to any institution." In the same meeting, a motion to "extend the course of the training school from two to three years . . . was carried unanimously."[20]

Clearly, much depended on the women who came to learn nursing, not only in 1892, but throughout the existence of the training program. Realizing this, Mrs. Bradbury and succeeding superintendents probably took some comfort in knowing that the decision to become a St. Luke's nurse was not hastily made. The mean time from when the nurses applied to the hospital and when they entered was approximately three and three-quarter months. This reflects a gradual increase from a low of three months during the first years of the program to nearly four and one-half months in the latter years.[21] Moreover, as the program matured, a larger and larger percentage of those who came for training were friends or relatives of nurses who had previously trained at St. Luke's.[22]

School officials certainly knew a great deal from reading their applications and letters of reference. Candid and often passionate descriptions about nursing and the women who sought to enter this field were the norm, in sharp contrast to today's tendency in discussing students to "bleach the intensity and directness from our language."[23] Additionally, many of the prospective nurses met with the superintendent for an interview. Such information gave Superintendent Bradbury, and subsequent officials, a surprisingly clear, initial impression of what an applicant was like and a sense of how well she would perform in training. Taken as a whole, the application records also provide an invaluable glimpse into the nature of nursing that spans four decades.

ESSENTIALS

All of the applicants who entered St. Luke's were women, and all were white. For the most part, they had never been married and, as the women assured hospital officials, they were "free from domestic responsibilities."[24] Undoubtedly, such characteristics reflect more about assumptions involving gender and nursing during this period than they do about official, written policy.

To begin with, training school rules did not specifically exclude men. Nor were applicants asked to list their gender. Instead, it was assumed that only women would apply. As the instructions about clothes indicate—"bring . . . two or three gingham or calico dresses"—men were not even considered as applicants. Yet the concept of nursing as an exclusively female endeavor took hold in Western society only in the last part of the nineteenth century. Prior to that time, men were an integral part of nursing's presence, performing the work of nursing in varied public contexts. Indeed, men often predominated in providing general hospital nursing, religious nursing and military nursing.[25] However, a resolute, Victorian reformer had other plans.

Florence Nightingale was determined to redefine nursing as a respectable occupation for women, a radical change in thinking that depended on a vision of nursing as wholly within a woman's scope of understanding and responsibility.[26] Any other vision would threaten the nineteenth-century belief in separate male and female spheres of activity and would doom the transformation that Nightingale hoped to achieve. Once accepted, the claim that nursing was rightfully a female activity meant that only women could be nurses.

For Nightingale, arguing that women were rightfully or uniquely qualified to do nursing was also intended to ensure a measure of independence from men in the medical/hospital bureaucracy. "There must be a clear and recorded definition of the limits of these two [male medical and female nursing] classes of jurisdiction" because, as she reasoned, "a man can never govern a woman."[27] In summing up her work, Nightingale stressed, "The whole reform of nursing both at home and abroad has consisted of this. To take all power out of the hands of men and put it into one female trained head and make her responsible for everything regarding internal management and discipline being carried out. Don't let the Doctor make himself the Head Nurse and there is no worse Matron than the Chaplain."[28]

Beginning with her success in introducing women to battlefront nursing, during the Crimean War of 1853, Nightingale's efforts threw open the door to paid nursing for increasing numbers of women, while closing this field to most men. Throughout the period of St. Luke's, then, the numbers of men in nursing nationwide remained small, with only a handful of programs preparing all-male classes for work in specialized areas such as psychiatry. Even this small percentage showed a decline. In 1910, for instance, 2.4 percent of all "trained nurses" were men and 6.7 percent of "untrained nurses" were men. Notably, the census definition of trained nurse included graduates as well as those in training. By 1940, the percentage of men had declined even further, to 1.8 percent trained and 1.0 percent untrained.[29] These figures leave little doubt that nursing had evolved in such a manner that, with few exceptions, only women were considered to be suitable candidates.

There was also no overt exclusion of persons of color at St. Luke's. Yet just as tacit restraints barred men from entering training, except in the separate programs established for them, so persons of color were silently barred from entering most training programs, including St. Luke's. Segregation of men and persons of color was simply assumed during this period. A noted historian on race and nursing affirms, "Hospitals and nursing schools followed the segregated pattern, which forced the establishment of hospitals and schools of nursing for Blacks. Black codes were set up in the South by law and in the North by custom."[30]

Applicants to St. Luke's were not asked openly about their race until 1920, at which time a one-word question, "Color?" was added to the application form. The women's responses indicate that they misunderstood what was being asked—typical answers included "medium light," "blonde," and "brunette." There is no evidence, however, that blondes were chosen over brunettes, or that any similar type of preference was enforced. Yet the written records, pictures, and interviews clearly show that only Caucasian individuals were admitted for training, emphasizing that underlying assumptions about race, rather than stated rules, precluded anyone who was not white from applying to the program. The only persons of color admitted to St. Luke's, as duly noted in the hospital register, were "colored patients."[31]

An example from the minutes of the Ramsey County Graduate Nurses' Association, an organization in which St. Luke's nurses played an active

role, illustrates the prevailing attitude toward race. It involved a request by
"Miss Benjamin, a (nursing) graduate of New York Hospital," to join the
association.[32] Such requests were taken seriously, due to the association's
control and operation, from the late 1890s until 1940, of the nurses' registry, the principal referral agency in the St. Paul area for women doing private-duty nursing. Local nurses claimed this as "the first official registry in
the United States established . . . by a representative group of graduate
nurses . . . solely for the mutual benefit of the group."[33] During this time,
private duty was the main source of employment for nurses.

For most nurses, including Miss Benjamin, private duty involved a system of work in which women were essentially independent contractors,
hired to nurse patients in homes, or occasionally, in hospitals. The Nurses'
Association, by virtue of its oversight of the registry, was a key organization
for nurses who sought work in the city and its environs. In this context, the
members of the association met to consider Miss Benjamin's request to
join them, on April 6, 1903.

Miss Benjamin's acceptance seemed assured. After all, she was a graduate of New York Hospital, which at the time ran one of the most highly
regarded training schools in the nation. The association regularly admitted
members from other states, based on the reputation of their training program. What made this situation different, however, is that members were
"considering the question of admitting . . . a colored nurse." Miss Benjamin's case prompted "considerable discussion," unlike other entries in the
minutes that indicated most issues were dealt with matter-of-factly and
with minimal discussion. The immediate response was, "We could not possibly admit her into full membership."[34]

Further proof of the problematic nature of Miss Benjamin's request
came when members were unable to decide about granting even provisional membership and "the matter was laid on the table." At the next
meeting, "the matter of admitting the colored nurse was brought up and
discussed" once again. This time the possibility of provisional membership
was not even considered. In their final statement on the issue, "it was
decided not to admit her."[35] As at St. Luke's, there was no written policy
against admitting African American nurses to the association, although it
was assumed that this would not occur.

~

All of the prospective nurses were asked about their marital status (see figure 2). But the question they were asked, "Are you single or a widow?"
revealed certain assumptions. Other choices such as married, separated, or

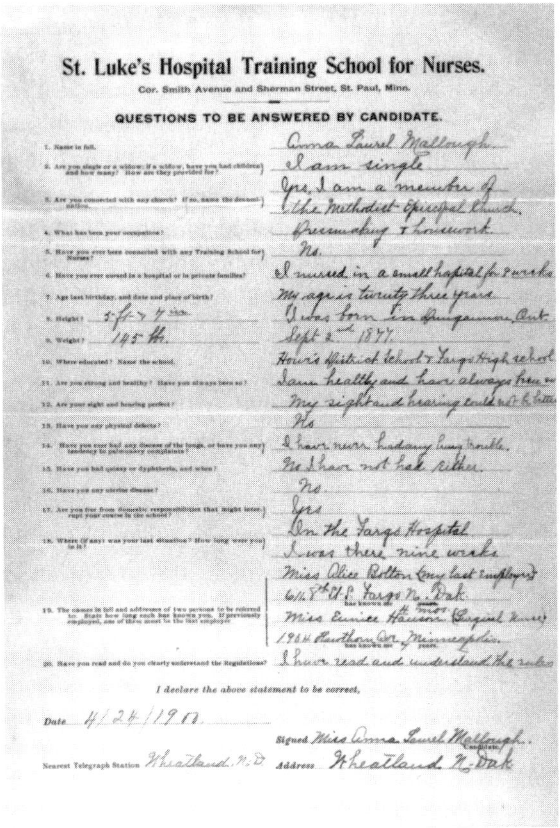
St. Luke's Hospital Training School for Nurses.
Cor. Smith Avenue and Sherman Street, St. Paul, Minn.

QUESTIONS TO BE ANSWERED BY CANDIDATE.

1. Name in full. Anna Laurel Mallough.
2. Are you single or a widow; if a widow, have you had children and how many? How are they provided for? I am single
3. Are you connected with any church? If so, name the denomination. Yes, I am a member of the Methodist Episcopal Church.
4. What has been your occupation? Dressmaking & housework.
5. Have you ever been connected with any Training School for Nurses? No.
6. Have you ever nursed in a hospital or in private families? I nursed in a small hospital for 9 weeks
7. Age last birthday, and date and place of birth? My age is twenty three years. I was born in [illegible], Ont. Sept 2nd 1877.
8. Height? 5 ft & 7 in
9. Weight? 145 lbs.
10. Where educated? Name the school. [illegible] District School & Fargo High school
11. Are you strong and healthy? Have you always been so? I am healthy and have always been so
12. Are your sight and hearing perfect? My sight and hearing could not be better
13. Have you any physical defects? No
14. Have you ever had any disease of the lungs, or have you any tendency to pulmonary complaints? I have never had any lung trouble.
15. Have you had quinsy or dyphtheria, and when? No I have not had either.
16. Have you any uterine disease? No.
17. Are you free from domestic responsibilities that might interrupt your course in the school? Yes
18. Where (if any) was your last situation? How long were you in it? In the Fargo Hospital I was there nine weeks
19. The names in full and addresses of two persons to be referred to. State how long each has known you. If previously employed, one of these must be the last employer. Miss Alice Bolton (my last employer) 614 8th St. S. Fargo N. Dak. has known me [illegible] Miss Eunice [illegible] (Surgical Nurse) 1904 Hawthorne Av. Minneapolis. has known me 7 years.
20. Have you read and do you clearly understand the Regulations? I have read and understand the rules

I declare the above statement to be correct,

Date 4/24/1900

Signed Miss Anna Laurel Mallough. Candidate.

Nearest Telegraph Station Wheatland, N. D. Address Wheatland N. Dak

Figure 2. Completed Application Form, Anna Mallough, 1900. From Minnesota Historical Society's Collection #152.K.20.7(B), Box 1, St. Luke's Hospital Records, St. Luke's Hospital Training School for Nurses, Folder: Anna Mallough.

divorced were not included. Quite simply, paid work was viewed as something that existed for most women only until marriage, and divorce or separation were unfortunate occurrences that shrouded individuals with suspicion.[36] As expected, then, the vast majority (97 percent) of trainees had never been married. However, there were exceptions.

An additional small percentage (1 percent) were widows. More surprisingly, slightly more were divorced or separated.[37] While the latter figure may not have represented a serious challenge to social convention, nonetheless, it demonstrates the willingness of training school officials to make exceptions to requirements. Still, the decision to admit a woman who was divorced or separated required a careful explanation. Thus, a nurse who entered St. Luke's in 1931 wrote, "At the age of eighteen, in 1923, I married a boy of twenty. The home of my dreams never came true. We went to live with his folks. I found I had jumped from the frying pan into the fire. Two years later my husband left. I did not know his whereabouts nor when he would return ... my husband was everything but a gentleman. He cannot properly support himself. I obtained my divorce on the grounds of cruel and inhuman treatment."[38] Satisfied with this description, and perhaps touched by the applicant's vulnerability and pain, the superintendent of nurses responded, "It would seem you have a just cause for a divorce."[39] An interview followed and the woman was admitted to the hospital for training.

For the superintendent, concern about divorce involved more than the moral implications of such a blemish to a woman's reputation. The hospital had a practical interest in making sure, as applicants were asked, that nurses were "free from any domestic responsibilities." Since the further a woman progressed in training, the more responsibility she could assume in her work, outside demands might result in the loss of an experienced worker.

This more mundane focus is evident in the situation of another woman who entered St. Luke's in 1906, after being divorced. She explained that she had obtained "an absolute divorce in the summer of 1901," adding, "It may be that I shall not be able to take the course, as I have a five year old son and it is not easy to arrange for a three years separation ... (but) I think I should enjoy the work, if one may use such a word in connection with suffering. ..."[40] Although the superintendent did not record any trepidation about the divorce, the nurse's admission was delayed until "a suitable home is found for her son."[41] In all, six women who had children were admitted. Similar to this example, they were accepted only after assuring hospital officials that their children had other, suitable living situations for the entire course of training.

Unlike divorce and separation, no exceptions were made for admitting married women. St. Luke's, and nursing in general, were not alone in this regard. "Bars concerning the hiring and firing of married women," as economic historian Goldin explains, "arose in teaching and clerical work from the late 1800's to the early 1900's."[42] In nursing, the prohibition on marriage was reinforced by irregular work schedules and the unique requirement, at once burdensome and beneficial, that women had to live in a nurses' residence during their hospital work and training.

Most remarkable in considering the gender, race, and marital status of applicants is how constant these remained over time. For more than four decades, nursing at St. Luke's was an occupation only for Caucasian women

who, with few variations, had never been married. Far from being u
this profile reflected general beliefs and standards, including the vie
paid nursing was women's work. These patterns were exceedingly in
tant in shaping the experience of nursing.

Like other occupations, including medicine, organized nursing was
emerging as a segregated field, a fact that would leave lasting scars and sus-
picions.[43] At the same time, nursing seemed destined to become an episodic
form of employment, a short-term occupation that a woman might pursue
before eventually marrying and raising a family. Equally far reaching, nursing appeared certain to develop apart from male-dominated power structures, a separation presaged by the ouster of the lady Board of Managers at
St. Luke's and sealed by the belief that nursing was the exclusive domain of
women. Yet aside from the inequities of gender segregation in limiting
nursing to women, the practice created an area of work in which certain
women-centered attitudes and practices might flourish.[44]

~

A close look at the applicants' ages reveals a pattern of change over time,
distinct from the consistencies just discussed. In accord with requirements
"universally adopted by first-class hospitals," the acceptable age range was
initially set in 1892, at "over twenty-one and under thirty-five years of
age."[45] By 1920 this was revised and women were told "there is no arbitrary
rule as to the applicant's age but preference is given to those between nineteen and thirty years." The age requirement was adjusted again in 1930,
with the stipulation that entering nurses be from eighteen to thirty-five
years of age.[46]

In actual practice, all of the requirements were used only as very general
guidelines. The youngest woman was admitted just short of her seven-
teenth birthday and the oldest when she was nearly thirty-seven. Still, there
was a steady decline in age over the three periods (see table 1). Various
researchers, working mainly from a premise of professionalization, link
this decline to the idea of perceived exploitation. Because of an increasing
scarcity of candidates, it is argued, hospitals were compelled to relax age
requirements in order to meet staffing needs.[47] However, the argument is
unsound due to a lack of evidence and, at least regarding St. Luke's, the suggestion of evidence to the contrary.

Changes in age at admission suggest that the program became more,
not less, selective in its choice of applicants. The average variance in age
among trainees dropped from four years in the earliest era to under two
and one-half years in the last. Moreover, there is no indication that St.

Table 1. Age at Admission

	Mean	Std Dev	Minimum	Maximum	N
1897–1910*	24.4	4.0	19.2	36.9	210
1911–1923	21.7	3.7	17.6	35.6	276
1924–1935	19.8	2.4	17.0	35.4	305

Source: Nurses' files from St. Luke's Hospital Training School for Nurses, 1897–1937.
*The time periods used in the tables and throughout the text were chosen for two reasons. First, researchers have asserted that policies of training schools varied widely based on who was in charge at the time. To adjust for this, periods of comparison were selected so that each spans the administration of at least four different superintendents of nursing and two different hospital superintendents. Individuals in these positions had the most direct influence on nurses' training. Second, the three periods bracket two of the most frequently cited reports involving health-related occupations during this era: the 1910 Flexner report, which studied medical education and marked the ascendancy of scientific medicine, and the 1923 Goldmark report, which was similarly aimed at professionalizing nursing education. Using the specified intervals of time made it possible to evaluate what effects, if any, these two events had on nurses' training at St. Luke's.

Luke's ever had a problem in attracting applicants. In 1893, for instance, there were 125 applicants to the training school. Of these, fifty were given consideration and twenty-five were accepted. In 1920, there were 117 applications and twenty-four women were accepted.[48] Applicant pools of this size would be the envy of most nursing programs today.[49]

Nursing fit within a larger context of gender and work. The decline in the age of entering nurses was consistent with trends in paid employment among women in general. In 1890, according to census data, labor force participation was 35 percent for never-married, white women in the fifteen- to twenty-four-year age group. By 1920, this percentage had risen to 47 percent.[50] Against this backdrop, there is scant support for attempts to link declining age at admission to arguments of scarcity or exploitation.

Yet trainees were generally expected to be in their twenties, not younger. According to usual interpretations, this expectation was premised on the belief that nursing demanded a high degree of maturity, which in turn was linked with age.[51] From the start of training, then, women had to manifest a certain depth of experience. Training could never replace this experience, only add to it. If such interpretations are true, women who wished to enter training but fell short of the age requirement would have argued for their admission in terms of unusual or advanced life experience. In March 1901, Anna Lucken made exactly this type of argument in a letter to St. Luke's. Though the ideal age for entering nursing at the time was generally con-

prove to be mature & age requirement is waived

sidered to be twenty-three, she reasoned that, "Although I am only twenty-one, I trust you will not let this bar me as I have been a teacher in the Public Schools of Wisconsin for five years and, being an orphan from childhood, I have seen more of the world and am older than most people at the age of 23 years."[52]

This argument based on maturity actually proved to be the exception. Other applicants took physical strength and endurance to be the important characteristics required, and made their arguments for early admission on that basis. Alma Strand's explanation in 1913 is typical. She pointed out, "I am quite strong. Have done quite a deal of heavy work and have always been considered strong for my age. . . . Tho I am not as old as the acceptable age stated in pamphlet (I) think I am as physically able as any one of that age."[53]

Those who wrote in support of the women used similar reasoning. One individual, a physician, intervened on behalf of an underage applicant by noting that "she is not yet 21 but her built [*sic*] is large and physically able to undertake the work."[54] A reference for another trainee asserted that "she will not be 20 till January, but (she) appears older on account of her well developed physique."[55] In describing a 1910 applicant, a nurse explained, "my little friend . . . is rather young being nineteen but (she) is well developed."[56]

Physical strength and stature were also used in making a case for the few women who exceeded age limits. In the hospital superintendent's interview notes from August 1904, for instance, the superintendent supported the admission of a thirty-six-year-old woman who was, nonetheless, "strong and healthy, young looking, weigh(ing) about 140 pounds."[57] As Floy Kellar summed up in a postscript to her 1917 application, "Please don't let my age count against me as I really am very strong and feel assured I can do the work properly."[58] Thus, in the minds of the applicants and hospital officials, age was mitigated by other, more important physical qualities.

High levels of physical strength and endurance were claimed by all of the women who entered training. Unlike with age, no exceptions or variations were allowed. In addition, the careful descriptions of physical attributes underscores how important these were seen to be for becoming a nurse.

"I have been thinking for some time of becoming a nurse," wrote Margaret Crowl to St. Luke's in 1900, adding, "I am well and strong and am confident that I can perform any work which might be assigned to me."[59] Her confidence was apparently well founded, because ten years later she became the superintendent of nursing at the hospital. Like Miss Crowl, a 1905 applicant asserted, "I have inquired into the matter carefully and am

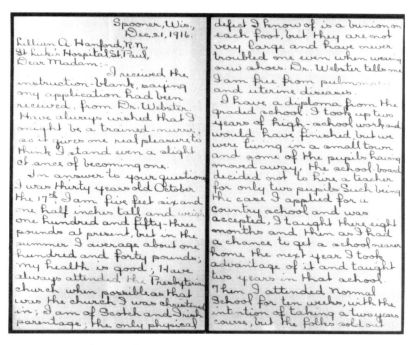

Figure 3. Excerpt from Application Letter, Ada Blake, 1916. From Minnesota Historical Society's Collection #152.K.20.10(F), Box 4, St. Luke's Hospital Records, St. Luke's Hospital Training School for Nurses, Folder: Ada Blake.

positive I have the strength to do the work required of me."[60] Two years later Susan Rightmire pointed out in her application, "I can walk a good ten miles or swim between four and five hundred feet without fatigue."[61]

These women were responding to the question, "Are you strong and healthy?" Sometimes this question was sent to applicants as part of a handwritten list of items to be answered; at other times it was included on an application form, and periodically it was brought up during face-to-face interviews (see figure 3). On the surface, it seemed to be a routine inquiry to which a perfunctory "yes" might have been the expected response. In reality, the women thought it worth answering with emphatic statements such as, "I never get tired," "(I) am very wiry and strong," or, as another nurse stated, "I have a strong back; I don't believe I have ever had a back ache."[62]

Detailed and impassioned responses clearly set apart the area of physical qualifications from other requirements for training. The women's answers also suggest that, at least in physical terms, applicants more closely fit emerging images of women's power than lingering Victorian notions of

feminine delicacy. This is illustrated in the following account from an applicant who was raised in an all-female household: "In 1913 my mother, sister,
and I took up a claim in northern Minnesota, just thirty six miles north of
Hibbing in the Bear River country. We spent practically three years on our
homestead . . . a great part of my time I spent hunting—getting all the wild
game we could eat. Partridge were very plentiful in those days. . . . On Saturday and Sunday my sister and I would take long hikes walking as many as
12 miles a day. When we proved up on our homestead and received our
patent from Washington, we moved back to Fond du Lac. . . ."[63] To the superintendent of the training school, this woman was "highly suitable" for nursing and so she was accepted without delay.[64]

Applicants and hospital officials were not alone in emphasizing physical strength and endurance. A recommendation for Ethel Burden, in 1904,
is typical of many others. Miss Burden was praised as a woman "capable of
. . . enduring severe tests of strength and vitality."[65] An 1899 applicant was
referred to the hospital in more simple terms, as a woman "not afraid to
work."[66] The preponderance of references to severe tests of strength and an
absence of fear about work is particularly noteworthy since these traits
were not mentioned in any of the training school literature. Apparently the
importance of such qualities in nursing was as widely understood to be the
norm as were gender, marital status, parental status, and age. Thus, a father
encouraged St. Luke's to accept his daughter in 1907 because, he stressed,
she is "strong in body being a little above the average girl in size."[67] In the
case of another applicant, in 1906, an acquaintance of the woman pointed
out that "she is physically wiry and possessed of large endurance."[68]

The theme of strength and endurance was repeated again and again
throughout the period of St. Luke's operation. In 1921, for example, a high
school teacher wrote about her former student, "I believe she should make
a good nurse. She is athletically built and seems to have unusual physical
strength."[69] Just over a decade later, a woman gave this plainspoken recommendation of her neighbor: "I think Marie would make a real good Nurse.
. . . [S]he is tall strong girl . . . and always willing to work hard."[70] Myrtle
Strand, one of the last individuals to become a St. Luke's nurse, was similarly described as "a large girl and of better than average strength and . . .
(thus) excellently qualified for nursing."[71]

These glimpses of individuals' applications and references offer insight
into the public perception of what it took to succeed in training, and thus,
what was truly meant by "a real good Nurse." Correspondents often linked
descriptions of specific persons with their ideas of nurses and nursing. To
them, "nurse" meant a woman who was capable of doing strenuous, physical work.

This image seems at odds with "the polarities which are broadly equated with masculinity and femininity."[72] In this industrial era, heavy, highly physical work was associated with men. "Light work" was considered the domain of women. As a labor lawyer stressed in defending special protection for women workers in 1916, "Women are more delicately organized than men."[73] It was by arguing for women's limitations that health and safety policies were first established; once established, they were later extended to all workers.

Feminist researchers point out, however, that such distinctions are less likely to actually operate in areas of work dominated by women.[74] Once a field of work is solidly defined as male or female, its tasks can still be seen as involving heavy and light work. Nursing was no exception. The acceptance of these distinctions, despite occupational realities, helped to define the wider, public image of occupations. "Gender . . . shapes what is noticed about jobs and the people who fill them," explains sociologist Steinberg. For example, in another industry—the female-dominated clothing and textiles industry—women have often been required to lift considerable weight, yet that requirement did not change the gender identity of the workers. Instead, clothing and textiles work was defined by its more "appropriately female . . . fiddly and sedentary" demands.[75]

In like manner, nursing retained an aura of femininity based on notions of women's predilection for nurturing or (the other side of the coin) their restriction to domestic personal service. The common perception among St. Luke's prospective nurses and their supporters seems to have been that nursing was characterized, above all else, by its physicality. This perception sidestepped the image of frailty associated with upper-class femininity and addressed squarely the real work required.

Even very public contradictions involving femininity, masculinity, and nursing tended to be tolerable. For instance, a physician gave legislative testimony in 1921 to support the argument that women make better nurses because "they sit up better and endure better."[76] If truly understood that way by society in general, then that superior endurance of women might somehow have helped them extend themselves into male-dominated areas of work, but such circumstance was rare in the period under study. Nor were stereotypical notions of men and women questioned when, in reporting on "the famous Red Cross parade of May 18, 1918," the *New York Evening Mail* glorified the Minnesota contingent of nurses in the parade for "averag(ing) in physique well above the army requirements for infantry men and . . . march(ing) like veterans."[77] This high praise for the women was actually *because of* their masculine attributes, but acceptable because it was within a feminine occupational context.

Any characteristic, whether consistent or contradictory, can become identified with an occupation's interpretation in society—how it is perceived—as well as with its reality. When seen through the lens of professionalization, the extraordinary emphasis on physical strength and endurance perceived by many in turn-of-the-century nursing suggests an exploitive system of work and training similar to that experienced by many male industrial workers. As nurse historian Ashley remarks, "Walking many miles in our white shoes, we were cast in the role of beasts of burden." "Rampant exploitation," she concludes, "prevent(ed) the intellectual development of nurses."[78] Of course, the perspective of nursing as a longstanding craft is no less powerful in influencing how and what is noticed about this field. Physicality and craft go hand in hand, so the prevalence with which nursing was viewed as a craft among the women of St. Luke's seems reasonable, not exploitive.[79]

Regardless of interpretation, however, the difficult, physical demands of nursing might have been the only option available to the women of St. Luke's. To explore this possibility requires a further look at their backgrounds, including where they came from, previous training and education, and work experience. Such exploration will also bring us closer to understanding the importance of the varying ways of looking at nursing's past.

Rural Beginnings

The women of St. Luke's were predominately native-born Midwesterners, with most (85 percent) originating from Minnesota or the four surrounding states. At the time they entered training, more than 90 percent also resided in this predominantly rural region.[80] This information alone suggests a less urban background than the nurses of the Northeastern Seaboard, the area covered by the best-known studies of nursing history.[81]

In Minnesota, settlements of 10,000 or more people covered less than 1 percent of the land mass during the entire first quarter of this century.[82] The region in general, and Minnesota in particular, were synonymous with rural and small-town living. In fact, the modest towns and sparsely populated areas from which many of the St. Luke's nurses came are a major source of America's rural mythology. Edward Eggleston's 1873 novel, *The Mystery of Metropolisville,* was set in the sleepy Minnesota town of Canon City.[83] One book in the *Little House on the Prairie*'s series was based on life in the area of Walnut Grove, Minnesota.[84] Small-town Minnesota achieved national notoriety with the 1920 publication of Sinclair Lewis's *Main Street,* while the bucolic image of the region lives on today in Garrison Keillor's popular radio tales of Lake Wobegon.[85]

'ty of individuals who entered St. Luke's to become nurses
ᴐse links to the agrarian and country life of the region. This
the analysis of the women's birthplace and address just
..aining. While small towns and rural areas consistently provided
...ie majority of trainees, the trend was decidedly rural. The percentage of
nurses who were born in rural areas increased from 37 percent to 59 percent between the beginning and end of St. Luke's training program.[86] In
contrast, Reverby's study in a different region—Boston's training
schools—for roughly the same period (from the late 1800s to 1939)
showed fewer and fewer nurses born in rural areas.[87] The difference is probably connected to the age of a region's settlement—its relative urbanity or
the rate of decrease in rurality—or to the development of other economic
opportunities for young women.

The rural ties of the St. Luke's nurses did not diminish over time.
Instead, the percentage of women who lived in rural areas just prior to
training almost doubled in the forty years between 1897 and 1937.[88] Thus,
when the leading newspaper of the region, the *Pioneer Press*, announced
"crops excellent . . . wheat acreage increases from 10 to 80 per cent . . . farm
hands are needed," as it did on July 7, 1918, no doubt most of the nurses
would have felt an instinctive sense of relief, being tied in to the agricultural well-being of the region.[89] In the same way, widespread feelings of
concern were likely evoked by the February 1931 "dry winter" prediction of
"a crop scare of no ordinary magnitude."[90]

Various historians claim that rural women were actively sought after by
hospital training programs. Reverby notes, for example, how one applicant
to a Boston hospital was praised for being from "sound country stock."[91] Yet
empirical findings fail to support the suggestion that concerted efforts were
made to recruit rural women. At St. Luke's, at least, no special preference
was expressed for nonurban women. However, important changes outside
the hospital certainly encouraged the shift toward increasing numbers of
rural applicants to become nurses.

At the opening of the century, travel from outlying areas to the city
could be a formidable undertaking. One nurse who arrived at St. Luke's in
1900, from just north of the Minnesota border, wrote in advance, "The
journey is so long. . . . God willing, I will be at the Hospital to go on duty
at the time stated."[92] The railroad had not yet extended to her area, so getting to faraway St. Paul meant several days of travel, first by wagon on
deeply rutted roads, next by train, then by streetcar, and finally, on foot.

Over the next several decades, however, dramatic improvements in
transportation made travel much less burdensome, bringing the entire
nation much closer together. Nowhere were these improvements more

striking, however, than in the relatively far-flung reaches of the Upper Midwest. Major progress initially came with the expansion of the three overlapping, fan-shaped sets of rail lines that spread across Minnesota and the surrounding region. Between the late 1800s and the 1920s, the network of railroads in Minnesota increased from 2,000 miles of track to more than 9,000 miles.[93] One set of lines extended into Minnesota from the preeminent transportation hub of Chicago. The second radiated out from Duluth-Superior, serving the northern forest and mining industry. The third set reached to the most far-flung parts of the region, from the historic head of Mississippi riverboat navigation at the port of St. Paul.

On the heels of rail development came the push to expand and improve the system of roadways. Early milestones in this undertaking included the creation of the state highway commission in 1905, a subsequent increase in the state road tax, and the passage of the federal aid road act in 1916 to improve rural roads.[94] By the 1920s, a swelling fleet of cars and trucks was rapidly replacing horses, wagons, and buggies, both within and outside the city. These changes literally paved the way for rural women to seek opportunities in the city, including nurses' training.

With obstacles to travel diminishing, the women of St. Luke's seldom wrote about their journey to the hospital after 1910. But the revolution in transportation not only provided the means for increasing numbers of women to come to St. Luke's, it also spurred changes in farming that compelled scores of potential wage earners to look elsewhere for work opportunities. One of the most profound changes—the replacement of horsepower by tractors—increased average farm size two to three times during the first part of the century. With the number of farms drastically reduced, more than half the farm labor force shifted to nonfarm jobs.[95] While some went into a few newly created occupations that allowed them to find work at home, such as providing services in tourism resorts, many of these individuals, women and men, looked to the burgeoning cities of Minneapolis and St. Paul for their livelihood.[96]

Adding to the rural exodus was a rural depression between 1919 and 1929. Two-thirds of the value of Minnesota farm crops was lost. Total farm value plummeted during these years of recession and depression, from approximately $500 million to $300 million. Minnesota was one of seven states that suffered nearly half of all the bank failures in the United States during the 1920s.[97] The effects of the economic downturn were widespread nationally but rural midwesterners were especially hard hit. With their already limited opportunities further constricted, nursing became an attractive alternative to young rural women.

"There was no money to do other things," explained one nurse who came to St. Luke's in 1926 from rural Wisconsin. She added, "I wanted to be a children's librarian."[98] Yet that would have necessitated paying college tuition plus room and board. Not only were her room and board taken care of at the hospital, but trainees were also paid a small "allowance" or stipend. Nursing was an attractive and respectable option. Still, nursing was beyond the means of those in the most desperate circumstances, since the stipends did not equal what they could earn in a real job (one where they were not "trainees" for two to three years). Furthermore, the small payments to trainees were under attack by national nursing leaders who argued that prospective nurses should pay tuition rather than be paid themselves, so there was no guarantee the system would continue.

Nursing leaders reasoned that requiring tuition and eliminating stipends would help to bring nursing into line with more academically oriented fields, such as medicine. Aided by hospital self-interest, their efforts led to a decrease, and in some places the elimination, of payments to trainees.[99] At St. Luke's the stipend decreased from a high of $12.00 per month, paid to "senior nurses" in the 1890s, to $2.50 per month for all trainees after 1910. However, the tuition idea was too extreme on top of the hard work performed by trainees. A token charge, in the form of a requirement of a $50.00 deposit, appeared in 1906.[100] The deposit was returned to the women upon completion of their training.

While changes in transportation and economics spurred the influx of rural women to St. Luke's, the steady increase was sustained by the close ties that were forged between rural communities and the hospital, based on personal relationship. For instance, eight women came to the hospital from a sixty-square-mile area in rural northeastern South Dakota that was centered on the small community of Bristol. This was one of the least populated areas in the entire nation. Yet such communities seemed to identify most strongly with St. Luke's. In contrast, only nine women crossed the river from Minneapolis to attend St. Luke's! As one woman from the Bristol area wrote, in recommending a 1916 applicant, "I think if you accept Lizzie's application you will find that she will sustain the record established by our girls at St. Luke's."[101]

Certainly the training program's solid reputation helped to win the dedication of certain communities, too. "One of the best" is how St. Luke's was described by the Minnesota Board of Nurse Examiners, a body which provided loose oversight of hospital training programs.[102] For the most part, however, St. Luke's solidity bespoke how typical and nondescript it was. St. Luke's graduates were well respected, although none achieved regional or national prominence. It was only one of more than a dozen hospital programs in Minneapolis and St. Paul in the first part of the century, representing a broad range of sectarian and nonsectarian interests. Other hospital programs operated in surrounding areas.

Plain but substantial, even St. Luke's physical presence, and its unimposing address on Smith Avenue, underscored the quiet respectability of the hospital and its nursing program. It offered safety to women who needed to look beyond their rural surroundings for work, during an era in which such an undertaking still seemed highly uncertain. Once women from a particular area started coming to St. Luke's, their advice influenced family members and friends to follow in their footsteps. The resulting bond between the hospital and rural communities, combined with the revolution in transportation and economic imperatives, ensured a steady increase in rural applicants to St. Luke's. It also ensured that others, such as the South Dakota woman quoted above, would laud the records of the St. Luke's nurses from their region. As an individual from a farming area near Wells, Minnesota, explained, "Our people are proud . . . of the class of girls sent (to St. Luke's) from here and that they are making a good record."[103]

Good Sense and Practicality

The fact that so many of the nurses had rural beginnings in common should not imply that other aspects of their background were the same or even similar. For example, applicants' previous education and training suggest there were various paths into nursing. Between 1897 and 1910 well over half of the women (57 percent) entered St. Luke's without a high school diploma though, remarkably, in the same period 15 percent entered the hospital with at least some college experience.[104] One in five, however, had never been to high school. Not until 1917 did the training program even request school transcripts, at which time "a high school education or its equivalent" was simply listed as "desirable."[105]

As time went on, the percentage of women who were high school graduates or above increased substantially, from 76 percent during the program's middle period, to 97 percent after 1924. Thus, even in the program's final years, the lack of a high school diploma did not necessarily prevent an individual from entering training. Yet rather than suggesting the use of mediocre entrance criteria, the women of St. Luke's actually exceeded national norms. According to the public use sample from the 1940 census, which is the first in which educational information is available, only 45 percent of white women nationwide had completed high school.[106] This completion rate approximates that of the earliest cohort of St. Luke's nurses and it is still less than half the completion rate for those who trained at St. Luke's after 1924.

The steady increase in the nurses' previous education, over a forty-year period, exceeded societal standards and seemed unrelated to any formal changes in entrance requirements. It might have set a standard. In 1909, accrediting agencies recommended a high school diploma requirement. Moreover, the largest increase in high school graduates (33 percent) occurred prior to a major nationwide study of nursing education that was designed to galvanize support for improvements in training. A major rallying point of this study, published in 1923 as the Goldmark Report, was a call for more stringent, educational entrance requirements.[107]

Still, St. Luke's became more selective over time in choosing prospective nurses. Yet it did so according to its own schedule and circumstances, not as a result of official leadership. This increase in selectivity challenges the usual arguments that standards fell to pull in poorly prepared applicants. "Because of a (growing) need for nurses," critics charge, an already "exploitive system" intensified and hospitals allowed entrance to rising numbers of inadequately prepared trainees, including individuals who had little or no chance of success.[108] Simply put, "the pressure for numbers made careful selection difficult."[109] Not, however, at St. Luke's.

Admittedly, the need for hospital nurses was on the rise. In 1873, a relatively modest number of nurses worked in the nation's 178 hospitals, which included fifty thousand hospital beds. In 1909, many more nurses were required, as there were now 4,359 hospitals with 421,065 beds.[110] Yet the constant rise in the previous education of the St. Luke's nurses indicates that in at least one nursing program a heightened demand for nurses did not mean lowered entrance requirements. The question of exploitation in early nursing still remains, but it cannot be supported empirically with data on St. Luke's educational admission standards.

Changes in St. Luke's applicants' qualifications correspond with major initiatives of nursing's leaders in the early twentieth century, such as the Goldmark Report. Such improvements bolstered the claims to the professionalization so fervently sought by leadership groups, but St. Luke's statistics also included some difficult-to-reconcile numbers of applicants admitted without a high school diploma.

Both St. Luke's and nursing leaders agreed that "a high school diploma or its equivalent" was desirable. The national-level leaders—individuals such as Isabel Hampton, Adelaide Nutting, and Isabel Stewart—decried anything short of this goal. Those in charge of the training program took a different approach, making exceptions for applicants who fell short of this one standard, provided they satisfied underlying qualifications. For the women of St. Luke's, previous education was deemed less important as an indicator than were intuitively assessed characteristics such as "good sense" and "practicality."

In place of a high school diploma, for example, approval of an applicant in 1900 was argued for by an assertion of her "unusual degree of common sense."[111] From a similar perspective, Marium Dyer explained in 1903, "I finished the grammar [*sic*] school," adding that she went on to study music, painting, and history. Then rethinking these last qualifications, she acknowledged, "I fear these studies would be of little help." It might be this very comment that led the training school superintendent to conclude that Miss Dyer "demonstrated good sense" and then accept her into the program.[112] The positive relationship between nonacademic or common sense, and nursing, seemed equally clear to a high school teacher who provided this simply worded recommendation of a former pupil: "She is a High School graduate of fair scholarship and ordinary ability. I should think that she would make an excellent nurse."[113]

Even as levels of previous education increased, related descriptions stayed much the same. Prospective nurses continued to be praised for qualities that included "sound judgment," "a head full of good sense," or simply for being "sensible." At the same time, the academic abilities of these same individuals elicited phrases such as "fair school work," "fair mental," or this more cautious appraisal: "as a scholar she is not brilliant."[114] For some, this presented a contradiction. How could a woman be filled with good sense but, when it came to school work, possess only "fair mental"? For others, there was no contradiction, but a clear description of a solid nursing applicant.

Did excellent nursing require brilliance, or at least academic aptitude? Sharply contrasting views emerged in nursing literature. Publicly, these views were expressed in the two best-known nursing journals of the early twentieth century, *The Trained Nurse and Hospital Review* (*TNHR*) and the *American Journal of Nursing* (*AJN*). Typical of the former, one nurse wrote, "The practical aspect of nursing . . . must never be sacrificed in the struggle after the more alluring and less substantial adornments." Removing any uncertainty about what she meant by adornments, the nurse dismissed higher education for nurses.[115] In contrast, *AJN* served as a forum for nursing leaders. In a characteristic article from this journal, two prominent nurses described nursing's "advance from the starting point of crafthood to journey's end—complete professionalization." Rather than eschewing scholarly pursuits, they emphasized that ultimate success for organized nursing depended on embracing nursing's "special intellectual concepts."[116]

Although separated by more than three decades, the two articles represent extremes in an enduring argument within nursing. The first, published in 1903, expressed the belief evident among the staff and applicants at St. Luke's that previous education was important only to the extent that it demonstrated an applicant's common sense. Although a high school diploma was desirable, there was no conflict in accepting a woman who lacked this credential, provided that she demonstrated her reasonableness through other efforts.

The second article, published in 1936, stated the position of a relatively small but visible nursing elite that was convinced that progress in nursing depended on more formal education, and particularly on a scholarly focus on nursing's special knowledge. The influence of these women, sometimes referred to as nursing's intelligentsia, centered on a select group of training programs in a handful of cities, including Boston, Philadelphia, Baltimore, and New York.[117] In their efforts to advance their cause, these elite encountered stiff resistance from what one of them described as "the prejudice against higher education . . . present in many hospitals" and among many rank-and-file nurses.[118] Compounding this difficulty were lingering societal doubts about the possibility of there being such a thing as "too much book learning for women."

The majority of nurses, like those at St. Luke's, were separated ideologically and geographically from the major leaders in their field. Both sides agreed on the importance of education, but they defined its importance in very different terms. At St. Luke's, the emphasis on good sense and practicality applied not only to applicants' basic education but also to any additional training and work experience that seemed to demonstrate these basic traits desirable in nurses.

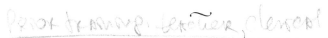

More than one in five of the women claimed previous specialized training, apart from grammar school, high school, or college.[119] Due to the gendered nature of paid work, this training fell into just a few categories for most women. Preparation for teaching was the most common, ranging from 37 percent of all additional training before 1910, to 46 percent during the last decade of the St. Luke's program. There was a range of variation in that preparation. Some women reported merely taking several courses over a single summer, often in their own high school, in order to qualify for teaching. Others completed a two-year program in a normal school or teacher's college. Regardless of the exact length of training, most were directed toward teaching in the elementary grades, in farm neighborhoods the same as or similar to their own, where there was a demand for female teachers. Such communities could pay women considerably less than their male peers would cost, with the result that 85 percent of teachers in Minnesota districts in 1906 were women.[120]

The next most common areas of prior training, clerical and nursing, also fit within the narrow scope of opportunities open to women in the early twentieth century. The two areas comprised approximately 20 percent each of all additional preparation. Most of those with clerical training reported taking a commercial course—one available for pay, outside of school—in order to learn skills such as stenography, typewriting, or bookkeeping. The women who described previous training in nursing usually were requesting to transfer to St. Luke's after the closing of their previous hospital program, which happened with increasing frequency in the 1920s. On average, they brought approximately one year of experience with them to St. Luke's.

Although the number of applicants who took commercial courses steadily decreased, there was a sharp increase in the number of women with prior nurses' training. The drop in the number of women with clerical training corresponded with the decline in the age of applicants, suggesting that many of those who might have chosen a clerical path in earlier years were now entering nursing soon after high school. At the same time, nursing trainees in many hospitals were seeing their programs close, a result of the deepening economic depression. From 1929 to 1939, over five hundred nursing programs across the United States, and many of the affiliated hospitals, closed their doors as the result of financial problems.[121] St. Luke's welcomed women whose training has been interrupted "through no fault of their own."[122]

The remaining types of previous training included instruction in dressmaking and tailoring, first aid courses, fine arts courses, and preparation for social service work. Despite the diversity of these experiences, the women offered a similar argument in their applications to St. Luke's. They stressed the practical nature of their prior training, referring to their subsequent ability to find skilled work as seamstresses, home health teachers, or music teachers. Overall, the previous training suggests that many of the applicants had alternatives to entering the hospital. Of course, the alternatives were limited to a relatively short list of occupations available for women in this era, but it is noteworthy that they existed.

~

A look at applicants' work history provides an opportunity to more closely explore the types of experiences that they brought to nursing, as well as to further consider the issue of alternatives. Early twentieth-century job options for women were decidedly narrow, although increasingly women found ways into other opportunities. For instance, Minnie Fay Hession

licewoman in St. Paul in 1913. Although her position made her
she focused on concerns traditionally associated with a
ere of influence, such as working with domestic problems,
ance halls, helping runaway girls, and finding homes for
unmarried pregnant women.[123] Years earlier, Mary Frances Kordosky
bought, furnished, and sold apartment buildings in St. Paul; worked as a
railroad inspector; and, in 1923, became the first woman to serve as deputy
sheriff of Ramsey County.[124] Another St. Paulite, Anne Egan Forrestal, was
appointed deputy collector of the Internal Revenue Service in 1922.[125] This
same year Else Redeker Obst became the first woman to be elected treasurer of Ramsey County.[126] Also during the first quarter of the century,
Sophie Greve Kenyon worked as a St. Paul stockbroker, Clara Linz
Bermeirer published the St. Paul German-language newspaper *Daily Volks
Zeitung,* and area resident Grace Hodgson Flandrau wrote two nationally
known novels, *Cousin Julia* and *Being Respectable.*[127]

Unlike these women, though, the women who came to St. Luke's to
practice nursing could not be considered occupational pioneers. Yet neither were they strangers to the workforce. A sizable majority (59 percent)
held one or more paid positions prior to entering the hospital. Specific
totals ranged from 79 percent who reported previous employment during
the program's earliest years, to 59 percent in the middle years of 1911 to
1923, to 49 percent during the later years of the program.[128] The gradual
decline in previous employment reflected a similar decline in the age of
applicants, suggesting that younger women, particularly those in their
teenage years, were simply too young to have accrued the same work record
as older women. Nonetheless, significant numbers in all periods possessed
substantial paid work experience before arriving at the hospital on Smith
Street, suggesting a strong orientation to paid work.[129]

When classified by type of work, the women's previous employment fell
into three distinct social and economic categories: lower status professionals, primarily teachers; skilled workers, such as clerks, typists, and
"untrained nurses"; and laborers (see table 2).[130] From 1897 to 1910, the St.
Luke's nurses who reported experience as laborers were employed in
housekeeping, child care, or some combination of these. The only exception was one woman who worked as "a companion to a nervous lady." In
other words, labor for women continued the interpersonal relations taught
to girls in their families and expected of them eventually as wives. The
nature of women's work was changing from interpersonal to impersonal,
however. Nursing, according to a 1930 report by the Woman's Occupational Bureau of Minnesota, "offers to women a reasonable income and a
life full of variety, interest and usefulness."[13] The possibilities contained in

Table 2. Previous Occupations of the St. Luke's Nurses (in %)*

	1897–1910	1911–1923	1924–1935	All
Higher-Status Professionals	0	0	0	0
Lower-Status Professionals	22.0	23.0	9.4	18.5
Managers and Proprietors	2.9	0	0	1.0
Skilled Workers	54.9	58.7	51.2	55.1
Farmers	0	0	0	0
Laborers	20.2	18.3	39.4	25.4
Number of Occupations	173	191	160	524

Source: see Table 1.
*Totals are based on occupational information from 684 nurses. For a detailed expla-
nation of the occupational classification used here see Olson, "The Women of St.
Luke's and the Occupational Evolution of Nursing, 1897–1915," *Mid-America: An Historical Review* 73 (April-July 1991): 135–50.

this modest description, assuming its accuracy for the period of study, may
have particularly attracted laboring women.

For the approximately 25 percent who reported having been laborers,
trained nursing presented an opportunity to increase their status, both
economically and socially. However, the type of work reported in this category was undergoing change. By the middle period, one in five jobs
involved factory work, including work in meatpacking plants, canning factories, industrial manufacturing, and a luggage factory. This trend continued into the last period, with factory work comprising one in three
laboring jobs.

Not only did the nature of work in the labor category expand to include
various types of factory employment, but the number of jobs as laborers
claimed by applicants nearly doubled from the earliest years of the St.
Luke's training program to the last. This paralleled the growth of manufacturing in the Upper Midwest, particularly in Minnesota. By the turn of
the century, Minnesota led the nation in flour milling and related industries, while other food industries, such as meatpacking, dairy, and baking,
grew even more rapidly. St. Paul saw the rise of numerous other smaller
industries, ranging from tent and awning manufacturing to the production
of men's suits, boots, trunks, and valises.[132] These were not the same jobs as
men performed but it was the same production work, the same class identity, and the same variety of concomitant class issues such as wages and
conditions of employment.

Minnesota also led all states in the number of young women working away from home. In 1900, the figure in St. Paul was nearly 30 percent.[133] This figure continued to rise as St. Paul and Minneapolis grew into a major manufacturing center, especially in textiles, requiring "an endless stream of young girls" to meet the demand for labor.[134] Yet more jobs, and the fact that young women were rushing to fill them, did not mean that the jobs or working conditions were particularly desirable. The state's assistant commissioner of labor, Mrs. Perry Starkweather, described living conditions for the women filling these new positions:

> Usually, two, three and sometimes four, girls earning $5.00, $6.00 or $7.00 a week, working usually at the same place, rent a room together. For this they pay from $9.00 to $12.00 per month. . . . The girls pool a common purse for food, and by dint of strict economy they frequently bring expenses down so that for four girls it amounts to $2.00 to $2.50 per week. . . . The evening meal is usually . . . purchased on the way home from work and is apt to consist of a bit of meat, a loaf of bread, cakes and pies from the nearest bakery. . . . If she pays $1.00 to $1.50 for rent, allows $1.00 for lunches, puts $2.50 into the common purse for food at home and walks to and from her work, she has from 50¢ to $1.00 or $2.00 left for clothing. . . . There is as a rule no provision for sickness. . . . As for amusements, they are almost entirely lacking.[135]

At the same time that new opportunities emerged in manufacturing, other avenues, such as teaching, became less and less available to young, working-class women. The professionalization of teaching preceded the professionalization of nursing. By 1900, the Minnesota Education Association, the leading organization of state teachers and administrators, had set in motion a far-reaching plan to advance the preparation of teachers. The organization expressed particular concern about "the increasing demand upon the high schools of the state."[136] Their efforts eventually led in 1913 to enactment of the requirement that all high school teachers hold a baccalaureate degree. The Minnesota legislature summarily upgraded the state's six normal schools to four-year teacher's colleges, offering baccalaureate degrees with a concentration in education.[137] As positive as these developments might have been for the improvement of teaching, they effectively closed the field to many young, working-class women for whom a four-year college degree would have been an investment they and their families could not afford to make. When coupled with the decreasing age of applicants, the more demanding requirements for teaching explain the steady decline in the number of St. Luke's nurses who reported prior employment as teachers.

Skilled work was reported at a much more steady rate, with jobs in this area clearly making up an important source of employment for the women. Among the clerical and sales workers were retail clerks, stenographers, bookkeepers, comptometer operators, postal workers, and typewriters. Other skilled workers included a baker, photographers, dressmakers, seamstresses, a dental assistant, milliners, hairdressers and, the largest group, nurses.[138] Indeed, more than one in five of those who entered the hospital between 1897 and 1910, and more than one in ten in subsequent years, were already nurses, although "not fully trained" in terms of completing a hospital course.[139]

These so-called "untrained nurses" were nonetheless listed as nurses in city and county directories and according to the national census. Moreover, they referred to themselves as nurses. Most were self-employed in "private nursing," or private duty, as it was also called. In fact, this type of nursing was the mainstay of most nurses until the World War II era. Private nurses were essentially freelancers who were employed by individuals and families. In general, they attended to a single patient, most often in the patient's own home, though occasionally in a hospital.[140] A Minneapolis nurse described private duty as "a somewhat mystical" undertaking, in which skilled watching and endless patience were major requisites.[141]

Both the large number of women who came to St. Luke's with previous employment, and the type of jobs at which they worked, reflect widely accepted beliefs of the time about who should enter nursing. These facts also conformed to Nightingale's ideas about nurses and nursing following her experience in the Crimean War. "Working-class girls," suitably supervised and properly motivated, would make the best nurses, Nightingale argued.[142] Such women would cope best with what she and many others realized was often hard, physically demanding work.

Applicants to St. Luke's clearly understood that nursing demanded an extraordinary level of physical strength and endurance. "By comparison with the nurse," Smuts observed of urban teachers at the turn of the century, teachers "enjoyed excellent working conditions, short hours, and, with respect to physical strains, easy work."[143] Even those for whom teaching was out of reach might have found a less arduous occupation in clerical or sales work. A stenographer stressed this fact when she wrote to St. Luke's in 1918: "Probably when I tell you that I am giving up a position here in which I can make more financially than I can in nursing, one in which I have shorter hours and easier work, you will realize what (nursing) means to me."[144] Indeed, one study of gender and work during this era declares office jobs were "the best-paid and most prestigious of positions open to young women."[145]

This begs the question, why turn to nursing? Changes in the workplace were opening the way for increasing numbers of women to enter paid employment in a variety of service and professional positions. Most of the new opportunities were in areas redefined as "women's work," part of a system in which the gender gap in earnings was profound and women were excluded from jobs with the greatest promotion possibilities.[146] Yet the St. Luke's nurses did have other options, some of which offered advantages over nursing. Even if hardship, low pay scale, and frustration were the rule in most women's occupations, why would a woman choose work that seemed to exceed the rather bleak norm? To attract the women described here, nursing must have offered more than just exceptionally hard, physical work.

Perhaps the determination of the stenographer noted above arose from a religious calling. Spiritual yearning is regarded as a major underlying theme of early nursing. Familiarity and comfort with the interpersonal nature of nursing might have drawn some, or conversely, the prospect of training might have appealed to some as preparation for later married life. Other applicants to St. Luke's, especially those already toiling in factories, might have been drawn to nursing for mundane but reasonable attributes, including the promise of room and board ("full maintenance"), a modest stipend, and the possibility of greater earnings in the future. Some women might simply have wanted a change, which nursing, according to the Woman's Occupational Bureau of Minnesota, offered in relative abundance. "A recent count showed sixty different kinds of work" open to graduate nurses, the bureau reported in 1930.[147] Still others may have come to St. Luke's to postpone marriage and childbearing, or as alternately suggested by popular stereotype, to marry a doctor and advance both socially and economically.

Rather than being consigned to speculation alone, as so often has been the case, the stories of the St. Luke's nurses emerge in records that enable us to understand with exceptional clarity why they chose nursing. Answering this "why" is important, because it sheds light not only on the women themselves, but on the nature of nursing. In the next chapter, then, we continue to explore the motivation, images, and expectations of the women of St. Luke's.

3

Ready for Work

There is no question . . . about my wanting to take up the work. I
have done almost all ordinary kinds of work and a great deal of
it—it is no trouble for me to work hard, and I expect it.

—St. Luke's Trainee, 1912[1]

fter her interview with the superintendent of nursing at St. Luke's,
in May 1929, Lydia Sommerfeld was definite about wanting to be
a nurse. In the hope that a follow-up letter would improve her
chances of acceptance, she wrote, "I am glad I was at your hospital last week
and hope I will be accepted for I was very much pleased with the place. I
now have made up my mind to go to your hospital if I am accepted and
continue until I am through. I have set down my foot and said, I will go
through the 3 years regardless of what I meet and have to go through. . . .
If I cannot go to this hospital I will have to try at some other one, so I
wished you would answer right away for I am waiting patiently."[2] St. Luke's
had made a favorable impression on Miss Sommerfeld and, although she
wasn't aware at the time, she had made a favorable impression on the
superintendent. She was admitted the following September.

Of course, Miss Sommerfeld's resolve may have been spurred by the
looming economic depression, her application coming only months before
a second major stock market crash abruptly halted "the wild orgy of speculation . . . which has taken place in the last five years."[3] However, even after
the second crash, confidence remained high in Minnesota. The *St. Paul
Pioneer Press* reported at the end of October 1929 that "business conditions
in St. Paul and Minneapolis are good and in the country districts they are
far from bad."[4] Moreover, Miss Sommerfeld's letter, like that of the stenographer cited in the previous chapter, typifies the determination shown by
the women of St. Luke's.

Yet the question remains, what exactly motivated Miss Sommerfeld and the other women to become St. Luke's nurses? Conversely, what additional qualities, if any, were hospital and training school officials looking for in determining who was right for nursing? After all, it was far from certain that an applicant would be admitted. As previously noted, for example, during a typical year 125 women applied, fifty were given consideration, and just twenty-five were accepted.[5]

SAINTLY NURSING

A common interpretation is that women often sought out nursing as a religious calling (see figure 4). In the early twentieth century, explains nursing historian Boutilier, a woman's "willingness to give physical care to strangers was widely interpreted as a concrete expression of spiritual grace . . . (involving) an ideal of 'feminine' self-sacrifice and self-forgetfulness."[6] Nurses became "ministering angels" and "ladies of the lamp," strengthening the construction of nursing as a female pursuit.[7] According to the Kalisches, nurses' training set the religious tone through "a very peculiar," almost monastic system of instruction in the "mysteries of ministering to the sick," in which nurses' "actions (were) governed by the dedication to duty derived from religious devotion."[8]

Yet beneath the veneer of religion, these and other historians argue, the ultimate goal of this system was less than charitable for nurses and nursing. Instead, it was simply intended to provide "a plentiful supply of female nurses . . . submissive, hard-working, loyal, pacific, and religious . . . not to educate [them] for a profession."[9] The tacit relationship between a religiously inspired nursing and problems in achieving professional status comprises a frequent theme in discussions of nursing history. As described in another account, "an unscientific and saintly nursing" prevented nurses from "understanding (the) structural characteristics of a profession."[10]

"Saintly nursing," as an allegory for nursing's slow progress in becoming a full-fledged profession, rests on two important assumptions. The first is that women tended to enter training to fulfill religious yearnings, and the second that self-sacrificing women were actively recruited by hospitals. If these assumptions are accurate, the St. Luke's training program would be expected to exemplify religious portrayals of hospital service.

To be sure, the effort to build St. Luke's Hospital was sparked by a religious leader, the Reverend John V. Van Ingen. Moved by the death of his young daughter in 1855, the "tall, venerable man" stepped into the Christ Church pulpit on Ascension Sunday of that year and appealed to his Episcopal congregation to establish an orphans' home and hospital in St. Paul.

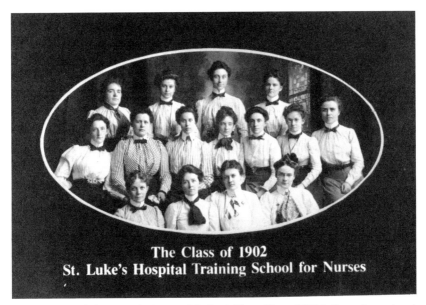

The Class of 1902
St. Luke's Hospital Training School for Nurses

Figure 4. St. Luke's Nurses in Front of Stained Glass, Class of 1902. From the authors' personal collection.

"Though I speak with the tongues of men and of angels, and have not charity," he exhorted, "I am become as sounding brass, or a tinkling cymbal."[11]

Van Ingen's appeal came at a time of massive change in the city, stimulated by the influx of new residents, nearly five thousand of whom arrived from other countries.[12] "Churches, which were everywhere in St. Paul," were on the front line of helping newcomers adjust to their new home.[13] The Episcopalians of Christ Church, whose slender "holy toothpick" steeple rose high on the bluff above the eventual hospital site, were eager to show that the city's Yankees were equal to other groups in meeting the charitable needs of those less fortunate.

The congregation quickly moved to support their leader's appeal for both the hospital and the orphans' home, marking the start of close ties between the hospital and the city's Episcopal community.[14] Their spirit of giving was both a sympathetic tribute to Van Ingen's daughter and a reflection of broadly based charitable sentiments being expressed in many of the other forty-nine congregations in St. Paul. As nurse historian Lynaugh points out, the founding of the new hospital likely drew strength from larger forces as well. During this era, "American Protestant denominations, such as the Episcopalians and the Methodists, saw hospital work as a powerful justification for their continuation in a period of increasing secularization and as a recruiting attraction for new members interested in charitable works."[15]

These factors seem to strengthen the relationship between religion and nursing, bolstering the perception that "religious imagery and exhortations to be 'otherworldly' permeated this field."[16] We expected, then, that the religious influence at St. Luke's would be significant and obvious, not only during training but also in the application process. In fact, however, the initial set of questions for applicants did not even inquire about religion. Well over one in ten (12 percent) of the women either failed to include their religious background in their applications (6 percent) or denied having any religious ties (6 percent).[17]

Beginning in 1897, the applications did ask women, "Are you connected with any church?" Those who answered "Episcopalian" actually comprised a small percentage of the nurses, considering the church's role in sponsoring the hospital. Their numbers ranged form a high of 19 percent during the program's early years to a low of 13 percent.[18] This might be consistent, however, with the fact that Episcopalians were a minority within the city and the region. Other mainstream Protestants such as Lutherans, Methodists, and Presbyterians predominated among the applicants, their numbers ranging from 49 percent to 68 percent of the total number of applicants. In addition, just as an absence of any religious ties was not an impediment to admission, neither was a more exotic religious background. Slightly more than 5 percent identified with religions that had only a modest presence in the region, including Jewish women, Latter Day Saints, United Brethren, Mennonites, and Christian Scientists.[19]

Only women from Roman Catholic backgrounds were underrepresented, comprising just 6 percent of the nurses. From its beginning, St. Paul maintained a predominantly Catholic stamp, with German Catholics settling in Assumption and St. Agnes parishes; the French Catholics near the Church of St. Louis; the Irish Catholics around St. Mary's, St. Michael's, and St. John's; and Czech and Polish Catholics near St. Stanislaus.[20] Most women from Catholic backgrounds who entered nurses' training in St. Paul, however, chose the program associated with St. Joseph's Hospital, the city's primary Catholic hospital. Catholic women were nonetheless welcome at St. Luke's, along with others whose religious backgrounds diverged from the hospital's Episcopalian roots. Even those who asserted "no religious affiliation" (also termed "nonprofessed" individuals) were accepted into training.[21]

Contrary to today's scholarly expectations, only four individuals said they chose St. Luke's because of its religious affiliation. This is all the more striking because applicants readily described a variety of other reasons for choosing the hospital, including positive experiences as a St. Luke's patient, the institution's location, and most frequently, knowing a St. Luke's nurse.[22]

Women doolud enter nursing because of religious motives

Of deeper significance, none of the women expressed a religious motivation for entering nursing. They focused on other reasons for becoming a nurse, such as the "need to be self-supporting" or the "desire to practice in all cases." The latter reason was given by an "untrained nurse," a woman with only informal experience in nursing, who sought to broaden her expertise and job potential. Like the decision to come to St. Luke's, however, the most frequent explanation for choosing "trained nursing" involved knowing a nurse or having prior nursing experience.[23]

Hospital officials themselves seemed to have little interest in applicants' religious yearnings. Unlike with essential characteristics such as age, applicants were not asked to explain or add information related to religion.[24] Such indifference to religious qualifications conflicts with the usual view of nursing during this era—as a quasi-religious occupation that was just beginning to advance beyond its saintly and self-sacrificing past. Findings from the applicants do not make sense within this paradigm, but closer study of what occurred more generally within the hospital helps to untangle the confusion.

By the early 1900s, hospital trustees and managers were charting a secular and pragmatic course for St. Luke's. In January 1903, a physician addressed the Board of Trustees and Managers "upon the urgent demand for additional accommodations in the Hospital to meet the constantly increasing number of patients seeking this as well as other like institutions."[25] He reminded the officials of a competing effort "by a committee of citizens, nonsectarian, to interest capital in a proposition to build and endow a Hospital, that should be Nonsectarian in character to meet the growing demands for such an institution."[26] The trustees expressed the concern "that for many years St. Luke's had been handicapped, as it was, from the fact of its being a Sectarian institution." The board then quickly moved to make St. Luke's "the nucleus of the proposed new institution" by authorizing its representatives to work closely with the group that had initiated the project.[27]

The board's success in making the hospital more inclusive naturally minimized religious influences. "When I came in '29," the nursing instructor in dietetics and hospital dietitian observed, "the hospital had been away from the church, that is the Episcopal Church. They called themselves . . . Protestant. And the then-rector of Christ Church said, 'The church didn't leave the hospital, the hospital left the church.'"[28] The patient census figures reflect St. Luke's effort to embrace the larger community. In 1920, for instance, just 6 percent of the 3,240 patients admitted to the hospital were Episcopalians, nearly the same percentage as Jewish patients (5 percent) and considerably less than Catholics (22 percent).[29]

Separation from church was quick
& painless

Episcopalians were a comparatively small group in the general community, as previously mentioned, so any plans to expand the influence of the hospital necessitated reaching beyond the bounds of a particular church. The ease with which this change occurred weakens arguments that tend to overemphasize the extent to which religion influenced hospitals and nursing. Loosening ties between St. Luke's and the church was not a soul-wrenching decision. No objections were registered. It was simply a pragmatic move, consistent with the low importance of religious emphasis among prospective nurses.

If saintly nursing existed more in interpretation than in reality, at least in St. Luke's and perhaps in other places like it, there seems to be little support for claims that a strong religious influence impeded nursing's professionalization. Still, making religion less central to discussions of the nature of nursing does not mean that qualities associated with wholesome and righteous living were of no importance. On the contrary, although religion invited only routine interest at most, training school officials were very concerned about an individual's moral character, as defined by societal norms.

Moral character was more important than religion

Moral character, rather than religious background, was considered paramount in selecting prospective nurses. Women were expected to be of "undoubted character," according to an 1899 description.[30] This was an expectation that remained constant throughout the training program's existence. Individuals were recommended with closely matched descriptions that extolled "an unsullied record . . . (and) exceptionally noble life and character"; "an unblemished Moral Character"; "good moral habits"; "character above reproach"; and "a very strong moral character."[31]

Explanations for the moral emphasis in nurses' training vary. One historian links the importance of moral character to Nightingale's close scrutiny of the moral background of those who entered the Nightingale School. He concludes that American programs "continued that moral tradition," in part because of nursing's reputation as a "morally dangerous" occupation.[32] Nursing, he reasons, put women in positions where they could easily be tempted by access to drugs and improper relations with men. Reverby takes a different approach. She explains that character was emphasized because it was seen as the essential skill of nursing. In the absence of other distinguishing characteristics, "respectability" had to separate the trained nurse from her predecessor."[33]

Moral prescriptions for nurses were similar to those imposed on single women in general, especially those seeking paid work. As Reverby acknowledges, educators near the turn of the century "were preoccupied with the molding of character."[34] The entrance of women into the labor force, in particular, raised concern about a threat to moral standards. Thus, at the same time "St. Paul women rall(ied) to the call for a great increase in knitting" to meet war-related needs in 1918, a national law-enforcement section was being created for the "protection of girls . . . flocking (to Washington D.C.) for government service."[35] A year later, social historian Arthur Calhoun warned that industrial employment threatened "to eliminate the truly feminine girl."[36] His warning was bolstered by an earlier report from the Minnesota Bureau of Labor that detailed some of the "moral perversions" that threatened women in the factory: " . . . the laxity with which clothing is worn, and postures are assumed, in the processes of manufacture; the constant association of both sexes . . . the temperature, excitement of emulation, etc., are all actively operative for evil."[37]

Others made similar warnings about women, not only in industry, but in the professions of law and medicine. One Minneapolis employer expressed the opinion in 1904 that women worked strictly for "the excitement, the opportunity for ogling customers, and display of cheap finery."[38] "A woman will sell her soul for a fine hat," worried a St. Paul newspaper writer in 1910.[39] Nearly half a century earlier, Jane Grey Swisshelm, noted Civil War–era "editor, lecturer, war nurse, crusader, and feminist" who lived and worked in Minnesota for some years, expressed similar concerns about "women workers." Too often, she explained in a letter to a Minnesota newspaper, the working woman responds to her male supervisor with "a 'prunes, prism, and potato' pucker, turns up her eyes like a duck in a thunder storm, or a juvenile bovine in the act of becoming veal, makes a pun and an impression . . . grows witty (and) tells the unfortunate man that she dreamed last night she was married *to him* . . ." (emphasis original).[40] Considering these long-standing, articulated fears about women in the workforce, the emphasis on morals for prospective nurses was not unique. It was consistent with the times.

Still unanswered, however, is just what constituted "character above reproach." The women's references help to explain. With some authority, a graduate nurse praised a 1910 applicant as one who "does not care for boys and is just the kind of a girl I'd like to have if I were choosing probationers."[41] Typical of most descriptions, moral character in this instance was connected to a woman's relationship with men. With only slight variation, a businessman recommended an applicant in 1915 by pointing out, "She is not one of the kind that go boy crazy."[42]

Over a decade later, in 1927, the message was the same, as a Wisconsin man confirmed that an acquaintance seeking admission to St. Luke's "has good moral habits and (is) not one that has chased the streets."[43] In another example, from 1928, a plainspoken father of an applicant wrote, "I have never known her to have any desire for bad company or vild partys [*sic*]."[44]

Also in 1928, the training program posed an additional question involving the character of applicants. The issue was not religious in nature; the program wanted to know, "Is your hair bobbed?" "To bob or not to bob! That is the question of the hour," proclaimed the *St. Paul Pioneer Press* in the mid-1920s.[45] Women who bobbed or cut their hair short tended to be seen as less strong in terms of character, interested in fashion and attracting men, certainly more so than in focusing on work. Therefore, the new question was aimed at insuring a nurse's "good moral habits," as understood for women in general during the early twentieth century. As another individual explained, in praising a 1932 applicant, "her morals are good . . . she is not an up-to-the minute flapper."[46]

For St. Luke's, the definition of moral character was specific and pragmatic. Women were expected to be morally unblemished, which meant being and having been prudent in their relationships with men. From the hospital's perspective, this definition was aimed at the factor that had the greatest potential to interrupt training and result in the loss of a worker, that is, the nurse's involvement with a man and the likelihood of marriage. In short, the hospital wanted women who were serious about nursing and who would stay for the entire period of training. Of course, St. Luke's was not unique in this regard compared to other employers or educators.

If nursing was not a special case, in terms of its religious or moral requirements, what does this indicate about the nature of this field? Abandoning claims of unusual purity or piety weakens an important aspect of the overall argument about nursing's supposedly uphill struggle toward full professional status. It also encourages broader comparisons and discussion, more closely connecting nursing to occupational struggles of women in general. Failing to let go of the rhetoric of saintly nursing and its suggestion that character, not skill, defined this fledgling occupation risks masking what nursing actually meant to those most closely involved—nurses themselves.[47]

PLUCK AND DETERMINATION

Moral character, although important, was actually part of a larger focus on a nurse's personality.[48] Like the comments on physical strength, the descriptions of personality were frequent, detailed, and emphatic. Two themes stand out in these descriptions: motivation and strength of will.

"There is no question . . . about my *wanting* [original emphasis] to take up the work," Alberta Wilson wrote in 1912. She added, "I have done almost all ordinary kinds of work and a great deal of it—it is no trouble for me to work hard, and I expect it."[49] This description, like those of others, underscored not only the strength and endurance of Miss Wilson, but also her willingness to do the hard work of nursing. Esther Carroll seconded this idea, remarking, "I am strong and very healthy. I can do good, hard work and am very willing."[50] In another example, from 1906, a married woman lauded an applicant for her motivation, while stressing her own ability to offer judgment: "There is one thing else regarding Miss Solberg (the applicant) . . . I consider it a matter of considerable importance in recommending anyone for such a position. I have had a good deal of experience with nurses having had six children and have been obliged to hire a great deal of trained help. Miss Solberg knows what it means to work. . . . And she has not done it with a long face either. I am so tired of people who work under compulsion. . . ."[51] There is no question about the attribute of motivation being emphasized in the above descriptions—what today might be called a good work ethic.

For others, the emphasis on motivation was stated more indirectly. "I take pleasure in writing to you in regard to one of our (Iowa Falls) girls," wrote Ella Hoag Crapset in 1900. "She is a faithful industrious worker . . . (who) will make an excellent nurse."[52] Willingness to do the work of nursing, implicit in this comment, was also apparent in the remark of a young woman who came to St. Luke's from Canada in 1910. She declared, "I am strong and healthy and . . . no stranger to work and I am not afraid of it."[53] A 1917 applicant provided this summation, "I fully realized as I became more and more interested in nursing that faithful and diligent application were the two great essentials."[54]

Along with their willingness to work, nurses were expected to possess another quality as well. This was expressed in separate yet similar praises, such as, "a strong and vigorous will"; "steady, level headed, and straight forward"; "a determined mind . . . an ambitious girl"; "very tenacious"; "pluck and determination"; "meets an emergency without panic or snap judgment"; and "not easily led."[55] These examples spanned the entire period of the St. Luke's program, highlighting that trainees were expected to have a strong will, the emotional counterpart of the program's emphasis on physical strength.

The importance that was placed on strength of will is best appreciated by examining some of the descriptions in greater detail. In 1917, for instance, an applicant wrote, "At the age of fifteen I was Club Editor on the St. Paul Daily News, holding that position until the fall of that year. . . . I gave a great deal of time to Asthetic [sic] Dancing and Sufferage [sic],

nging to the different Suffrage and Public Service Clubs. . . . I gave and
...ped in giving Red Cross lectures and organizing Red Cross Units. . . ." [56]
These experiences made up for being under the preferred age for this
period, since she was only eighteen, and for the fact that she did not have a
high school diploma. From the point of view of hospital and school officials, here was undoubtedly an individual with "a determined mind . . . an
ambitious girl."

Nor did the emphasis on inner strength change with time. In 1933, a
teacher insisted that a former pupil of hers would make an excellent nurse
because "she does not shun a front seat; moreover she always has a contribution to make to every class discussion. She is courteous, but never obse-
quious. . . . Although she does not flaunt her personality, both students and
teacher are agreeably conscious of her presence. Altogether she is a girl in
control of herself." [57] To the applicants, as well as their references, it was no
secret that nursing was a formidable undertaking that demanded inner
strength, being in control of one's self. Still, this picture of strong-willed
and motivated women is difficult to reconcile with the predominate view
that training programs were designed to produce "quiet, submissive
slave(s)," demonstrating "unquestioning subservience" and "docility." [58]

It is possible that St. Luke's was an exception to other training schools. As
previously discussed, however, St. Luke's found its place among hundreds of
other Midwestern training programs, as a respected but unassuming institution. From its early religious sponsorship and moderate size to its reliance on
apprenticeship labor, St. Luke's represented the norm for hospitals and training schools. Its reputation was one of providing "good training" in a "proper
hospital," no doubt necessary requisites for attracting a regular supply of
applicants. [59] And just as its opening was part of a nationwide increase, so its
closing was shared with a majority of other programs. [60] Even its nondescript
address on Smith Avenue served as reminder of the program's "solid nurses,"
none of whom would achieve regional or national prominence. [61]

What this strongly suggests, then, is inaccuracy in conclusions about
personality and nursing that are deeply rooted in portrayals of women as
weak and submissive. "The research (on nursing's past) resounds with the
words paternalism, submission and oppression," as one nurse observes. [62]
However, if prospective nurses at average institutions like St. Luke's—and
by implication nurses—are best described as motivated and strong, it
would be difficult to construct an argument for exploitation. An argument
for making use of nurses can be made, yes, but exploitation? It seems not.
This observation defies both the prevailing interpretation of nursing and
what feminist historian Scott describes as the "masculine/feminine . . .
opposition perceived as natural," according to which traits such as "ambi-

tion," "tenacity," and "determination," like physical strength, are used to typify men rather than women.[63]

But there is nothing to prevent individuals from reinterpreting existing definitions to explain their own situations, as Scott adds. Nursing may indeed have been one type of "situation" that prompted women to redefine themselves. According to nursing historian Melosh, "the literature and culture of apprenticeship . . . undercut cultural ideals by testing prescribed characteristics of 'femininity' against the demands of hospital life. As young women converted to the nursing creed, they came to see delicacy and refinement as mere squeamishness." [64] Such reasoning closely matches the thoughts and conclusions expressed by the women and their references. As a teacher explained in recommending a 1910 applicant, "She is ambitious, vigorous and energetic . . . so she seems . . . fitted to take up the arduous and trying things in a nurse's life."[65] This recommendation also touched on a view of nursing that persisted throughout the training program's existence, the "arduous and trying" nature of nursing.

~

"Many times during the past few years I have thought I would like to take the course of training for nurses," wrote Maude Mckay, a 1904 applicant from St. Paul. She went on to point out, "I have never been in a better condition to take up such arduous labors as I know this training will have for me."[66] Ms. McKay was well informed about what was in store for her at St. Luke's, as were most other applicants. For instance, a graduate nurse wrote to the hospital in 1910 on behalf of "a little friend who wishes to be a nurse." The graduate emphasized, "Vera is possessed to be a nurse. I explained all the disagreeable features and the hard work but she is still determined."[67]

For some, the hard work of nursing was an unspoken but implicit message. Consider again the determination of Miss Sommerfeld, the woman cited at the start of this chapter, who vowed to "set down my foot" to become a nurse. Her resolve "to go to your hospital . . . and continue . . . regardless of what I meet and have to go through" left no doubt that she expected nurses' training to make extraordinary demands.[68] Still, the applicants envisioned more than hard work alone. They expected, through an apprenticeship type of training, to acquire the skills of nursing and to become proficient in the use of these skills. Thus, they applied to enter the hospital rather than the school. They sought to learn "practical skills" while earning a modest pay.[69] And they asked to become nurses rather than students or student nurses.

"I shall be pleased," stated Eleanor Mallough in 1900, "to report at your hospital prepared for duty."[70] Her use of the term "hospital" rather than "school" was no mistake. As Lila Jarvinen explained in 1924, "I am interested in taking up nursing next fall, and for that reason I would like to get some information concerning your hospital."[71] Another applicant emphasized, "I am writing to get an idea as to which Hospital I would like to enter."[72] Of course, critics might charge that regardless of terminology, the women and their references still expected a customary academic setting. However, further exploration supports a different view.

"I know a good deal about the Hospitals of the City and I am confident that if Miss Price (the applicant) should be accepted as a Nurse, she will be an addition of importance to the staff and a credit to the institution."[73] This comment, written by a St. Paul man in 1901, is typical of others in the application material in that it was directed more at employment than study, at least in a traditional academic sense. Not surprisingly then, Lucy Baker did not ask to become a student when she wrote to St. Luke's in 1902. Instead, she declared, "I desire to be come [*sic*] a nurse in your hospital."[74] In another instance, a businessman who had recently learned of an employee's decision to enter St. Luke's observed, "You ought to be congratulated on having her as one of your nurses."[75]

With obvious knowledge about the functioning of a training school, Evalyn Schoch asked in 1909 "for a position as probational nurse in St. Luke's Hospital."[76] Probationer, or "probie" for short, was the commonly used term to describe a woman during the initial phase of training. Further undermining the idea that prospective nurses anticipated a classroom environment, Emma Man wrote in 1904 about her "desire to become an applicant for the position of nurse . . . (at) the St. Luke's Hospital, in oder [*sic*] to learn the work."[77] Eight years later, Margaret Crary expressed her hope "that I fill all needed requirements in order to be a nurse at St. Luke's Hospital."[78] Not only did these last two applicants use the language of work rather than study, but they directed their comments to the hospital superintendent, instead of the superintendent directly in charge of the training school.

Hospital superintendents were in charge of the day-to-day functioning of the institution, while superintendents of training were ostensibly responsible for the operation of the school. In truth, the two roles were constantly blurred, with the same individual often leaving one post only to assume the other.[79] Further highlighting the overlapping roles was the fact that the title of superintendent of training was used interchangeably with that of superintendent of nursing. In short, there was slight separation between hospital and training programs. As a result, applicants were as likely to direct their inquiries to one superintendent as to the other, with either superintendent responding.

There were questions from applicants about where to send applications and reference letters, but there was no uncertainty about key words used in these documents. When referring to nurses' training, "hospital" and "nurse" nearly always substituted for "school" and "student." The latter terms were consistently used, however, in referring to previous education outside the hospital. Applicants and their references saw a clear distinction between classroom learning and nurses' training. In the rare instances in which the term "student" was applied to nurses' training, the descriptions incorporated qualifying language. One woman, for example, requested to become "a student nurse on your staff."[80]

The essence of nurses' training was clarified by a high school teacher, who recommended a former student in 1931 as "excellent material . . . to serve three years' apprenticeship."[81] Of course, apprenticeship is usually viewed as extending beyond just a job to include learning by practical experience. This fact was explored in a recent study of gender and job choice near the turn of the century, which described the three types of occupations in the period. The first type included work that "usually required no experience," such as factory operatives. In contrast were jobs to which entrance was mainly determined by classroom education, including certain clerical positions. Between these two alternatives were skilled trades, positions that required individuals to serve an apprenticeship. Apprenticeship of steamfitters and plumbers, for example, involved four levels of practice, beginning with "inexperienced helpers" and progressing to "second men."[82]

It was this last type of occupation that was on the minds of the individuals who sought to "take up nursing" at St. Luke's. Thus, when Della Sweeney applied to the hospital in 1902, she did so to obtain "the practice essential for becoming a trained nurse."[83] Nearly thirty years later, a clergyman recommended a woman because, he explained, "I feel quite sure that Miss Turek [the applicant] will make a success . . . during her training and practice as a trained nurse."[84] These words—"training," "practice," and "apprenticeship"—filled the application material from 1897 to 1937, symbolizing the distinct expectations about nursing that were held by the women and their references.

Just what the women hoped to gain through their apprenticeship, if not scholarly satisfaction, was characterized by one individual in 1902 as "the important lessons for practical usefulness."[85] Others expressed similar ideas, including a postal clerk from Fairfax, Minnesota, who explained her decision to enter St. Luke's in 1912 by noting, "Have decided that nursing is the most practical work."[86] Further separating them from students in usual classroom settings, prospective nurses also assumed they would be paid while learning the practical skills of nursing.

Before she would consider entering the hospital, in 1900, Gertrude Westman wanted to know, "is the 1st year gratuitous . . . and what remuneration is allowed during the 2nd and 3rd (years)?"[87] Likewise, Clara Ball asked for information about "the requisite wardrobe (and) the wages."[88] At least twenty individuals made similar inquiries about the amount they would be paid while in training, which generally ranged from $4 to $10 a month depending on experience.[89] Only one individual inquired about an academic matter.

The view of nursing held by the women of St. Luke's, at least leading up to training, was certainly far from new. They believed nursing to be a demanding occupation, one that required mastering certain pragmatic skills during a period of arduous, apprenticeship training. Beyond nursing, their expectations fit the definition of skilled trades or crafts, areas of work, which traditionally "stressed the superiority of practical training over purely scholastic training."[90] Within nursing, there was a long tradition of apprenticeship learning on which to build.

A 1902 applicant to St. Luke's seemed to bridge the gap between the more informal apprenticeship in nursing, which took place on an individualized basis during much of the nineteenth century, and the more formal hospital training that came later. The woman expressed her desire to enter the hospital "in order to complete the instruction and practice" that she had already begun "as assistant to a well-trained and exceptionally good nurse."[91] She was accepted without question. Indeed, the most famous nurse to practice in the Minneapolis-St. Paul area never attended nursing school. Yet this did not stop Sister Elizabeth Kenny from adopting the British honorific for head nurse, "Sister," prior to her arrival in Minnesota and her founding of the Sister Kenny Institute to aid victims of poliomyelitis.[92] She had claimed this title after years of nursing practice in the Australian outback during the early 1900s.

A prominent scholar on "gender and the professional predicament in nursing," sociologist Davies, suggests that reliance on practical training or apprenticeship in nursing has its basis in the unique worldview of femininity.[93] This worldview derives from "a concrete and contextual cognitive orientation," in which knowledge takes on a provisional character. For individuals who approach life from this perspective, understanding must be confirmed in context and in use, experience must be coupled with formal expertise. Within the contrasting masculine view, Davies contends, knowledge is more abstract and fixed. It embraces "the concept of self as expert . . . knowledge as acquisitions, things that are displayed and can be put to use at will."[94]

Yet the feminine emphasis on experience and contextual understanding, and the relationship of these to nursing, are apt to be overlooked in a society in which the hegemony of masculinity tends to silence other ways of thinking and acting. "Your vision, extensive and expansive as it is," remarks Bologh in clarifying the masculine worldview of German sociologist Weber, "is the vision from your body, inscribed with your gender, your place, your time."[95] Bologh continues, "it may be the vision that enables you to make your way in and through the world; but it also restricts what you can see, what you can experience and what you know."[96]

Those who controlled the rapidly expanding hospital system, a group largely comprised of wealthy white men from the field of medicine, undoubtedly found the apprenticeship system of hospital labor to be economically advantageous. According to various historians, hospital authorities also saw this system as a means of maintaining social and intellectual control over the nursing profession.[97] Their interests frustrated repeated efforts by prominent nurses, including Adelaide Nutting, Isabel Hampton Robb, Lavinia Dock, and Isabel Stewart, to institute changes in nursing similar to those occurring in medicine. Such changes would have moved nursing closer to a more academic and expert-focused occupational model, consistent both with medicine and the masculine worldview described by Davies.

In her classic essay on early hospitals and nursing, Ashley concludes that nursing leaders "lacked a full appreciation of the extent to which more powerful male-dominated groups would attempt to stop their growth with little consideration of their ideal."[98] What she and like-minded historians seem to miss, however, is the depth of belief in a competing image of nursing held by prospective nurses. Nor is there appreciation of how this image may have been reinforced by a distinctly feminine way of knowing and perceiving the world. These are crucial factors in explaining the persistence of a view of nursing among entrants to the field that directly opposed the outlook of nursing leaders.

Still, the uniform perception of nursing among applicants to this field remains somewhat puzzling, if one assumes that prospective nurses came from different social classes. That assumption would be reasonable, given nursing leaders' recurring strategy for advancing nursing's professional status by calling for recruitment of a higher class of women and, at various points, the recruitment of men. Heeding such appeals, certainly some of the women must have favored, if not fully embraced, the image of nursing espoused by nursing leaders. The question is, did the call for higher-class trainees result in trainees of higher-class background?

A QUESTION OF CLASS

"The question of (nurses') social class . . . has been troubling at least since the early nineteenth century," observes one historian of nursing.[99] It was troubling indeed for early nursing leaders, who believed the issue of social class was inextricably tied to their struggle to carve out a place for nursing among the professions. They concluded that increasing numbers of trainees would have to come from middle- and upper-middle-class backgrounds, as was the case in medicine, in order for nurses to achieve their rightful place as physicians' colleagues, rather than handmaidens.[100] Nursing leaders rejoiced when the same conclusion was reached by May Ayers Burgess, a Ph.D. statistician who headed a national nursing reform committee in the 1920s and early 1930s.

Burgess sought to clarify the threat that existed to the advancement of nursing, in the form of women of "inadequate social and academic background."[101] Equating educational attainment and class, she declared that women from working-class origins should be discouraged from entering nursing because "these undereducated, unprepared women make trouble within the profession. Many of them are drawn from a social group which is not strictly professional in character. They are the ones who are talking trade unionism for nurses."[102] She pointed out that it was natural for these women to lean toward trade unionism because "their fathers, brothers, and sweethearts are ardent members of trade unions."[103] However, she continued, the end result is a group of individuals who "are less and less inclined to accept leadership from other nurses whose academic and social backgrounds are better."[104] Burgess echoed the thoughts of prominent nurses when she emphasized, "Somehow these undereducated women, in inadequate social and academic background, must be kept out of the profession."[105]

Writings such as those of Burgess, along with other scattered, anecdotal evidence, lend support to the idea that pressure to elevate the social class of nurses led to the development of a two-tier system of work and training. Historians surmise that nursing's elite—public-health workers, administrators, and educators—came from the middle class or above, while the majority of nurses had more modest backgrounds.[106] Most numerous in the latter group, supposedly, were women from families of farmers and skilled artisans. The St. Luke's records make it possible to explore the issue of class in a more systematic way and, in particular, to evaluate the success of leaders' arguments for recruiting a higher class of women into nursing.

Father's occupational information was available for more than four out of every ten of the applicants.[107] Although this is not a precise measure of class, it provides a useful estimate of the relative positions of the women

Table 3. Occupations of Fathers (in %)*

	1897–1910	1911–1923	1924–1935	All
Higher-Status Professionals	10.3	13.5	11.6	12.1
Lower-Status Professionals	9.3	6.5	4.5	6.6
Managers and Proprietors	24.7	22.6	24.1	23.6
Skilled Workers	43.3	36.8	28.6	36.0
Farmers	4.1	11.6	19.6	12.1
Laborers	8.2	9.0	11.6	9.6
Number of Fathers	97	155	112	364

Source: Nurses' files from St. Luke's Hospital Training School for Nurses, 1897–1937; city and county directories, census manuscripts.
*For a detailed explanation of the occupational classification used here see Olson, "The Women of St. Luke's."

within the social structure. "Rags to riches" stories notwithstanding, research into early-twentieth-century social mobility and gender demonstrates that a father's status, conveyed in large part by occupation, is "clearly transmitted to daughters as well as sons," . . . play(ing) an important role in offspring's occupational attainment."[108] This finding is crucial to considerations of class and nursing, because an individual's social position suggests shared dispositions, including similar views and attitudes about the nature of nursing.[109]

Close to two-thirds of all fathers with identified occupations were employed as skilled workers (primarily clerical and sales positions) or managers and proprietors (see table 3).[110] In this respect they were linked by a similar social position, generally regarded as below those in traditional professions and above laborers. However, while the proportion of managers and proprietary workers remained steady over time, varying by only one to two percentage points, the percentage of skilled workers gradually decreased. This was due almost entirely to a drop in the number of clerical and sales workers, a change that was balanced by a corresponding increase in farmers, from fewer than 5 percent during the earliest years to nearly 20 percent during the final decade of the program. This last change was consistent with the lack of economic opportunity for women in rural areas and the increasing presence of women from rural backgrounds at St. Luke's.

The percentage of fathers who were employed as higher-status professionals remained relatively small throughout the different periods. Moreover, in the last period of St. Luke's operation, the total in this category declined to less than 12 percent rather than increasing as nursing leaders hoped. Even this figure may be somewhat inflated, considering that applicants were probably more inclined to provide occupational information for a father who was a physician, clergyman, or lawyer—the main titles subsumed here—than for fathers with less prestigious work backgrounds. In any event, the percentage of fathers who were higher-status professionals represented a very small number of women. Yet it was this group whom the leaders of nursing deemed the best applicants, the ones most likely to share their vision of nursing.

An even smaller percentage of applicants were lower-status professionals, primarily teachers. The number of fathers in this category declined over time by more than half, suggesting that nursing leaders were no more successful in enticing applicants from families with this type of background than those from families of higher-status professionals. Indeed, lower-status professionals and laborers accounted for the smallest percentages of applicants. This last finding was particularly revealing because it differs markedly from the national statistics. Analysis of the 1910 Public Use Sample shows that more than 35 percent of nurses nationally had fathers who were laborers.[111] However, an important difference between St. Luke's numbers and the national totals is that the public use sample combined trained and untrained nurses.[112] Although nursing leaders apparently failed in their efforts to attract greater numbers of women from professional backgrounds into hospital training, it appears they might have had some success in discouraging recruitment of individuals from laboring backgrounds.[113]

The distinctness of the applicants' family backgrounds is highlighted by comparison with the occupational pattern of their references.[114] In each of three fifteen-year periods, 80.2 percent of the references came from the higher-status professional category. While 34.1 percent (just over one-third) were physicians and members of the clergy, a majority had other prestigious positions, including attorneys, school superintendents, business executives, judges, and bank presidents. A relatively small number were skilled and other similar status workers, mainly nurses. None were laborers.

This look at occupational backgrounds, more exact than in previous accounts, supports the idea that most nurses came from "modest backgrounds," although generally not from families of unskilled workers. The stability of this pattern further suggests that the persistence of a particular view of nursing was likely reinforced by the large majority of women who shared a common social position. There is no evidence from St. Luke's of attempts to change this situation by giving preference to applicants whose "social backgrounds are better."[115] Indeed, the small number of women from higher-status family backgrounds who entered St. Luke's were admitted precisely because they shared a common image of nursing.

Those accepted into training at St. Luke's saw nursing as an intensely physical occupation that demanded strength of will and emphasized the superiority of practical work and training over academic pursuits. In one sense, this image challenged stereotypes that ascribed qualities of strength and skill only to men, and reserved terms such as self-sacrifice, piousness, and delicacy, for women. Perhaps, as at least one historian has suggested, this prompted some of the women to redefine themselves.[116] Still, any threats to masculine stereotypes were mitigated by labeling nursing "woman's work," thereby removing the contradictions from close scrutiny. In addition, the emphasis in nurses' training on experience and contextual understanding—the essence of apprenticeship learning—may have been easily accepted and even welcomed by individuals for whom this type of learning was familiar and comfortable, part of their feminine worldview.

This same picture of nursing is seen by others as proof of a repressive system of work and training. Nursing leaders, as well as many historians of nursing, have been drawn to such a conclusion by their impression of the field as struggling for the same professional status enjoyed by physicians. In regard to class and social position, the assumption that this struggle had wide support led one historian to recently suggest that trainees "bartered transient workplace exploitation and devaluation for the enduring status and prestige their identity as nurses gave them in their communities."[117] To be sure, the women of St. Luke's, like apprentices in hundreds of other training schools across the United States, provided an accessible, inexpensive supply of labor to hospitals. However, the refrain of hardships and exploitation, with only secondary mention of benefits, differs markedly from the image of nursing held by ordinary women who sought to enter nurses' training.[118]

For women who were just emerging from the constraints of Victorian thinking, the turn-of-the century hospital training schools "presented the attractions of work outside the home."[119] These attractions included portrayals of female competence, commitment to work, and the means to independent support. Despite its faults, the hospital system of work and training was perceived by those who chose it as offering positive opportunities. Thus, with eyes open and a well-defined impression of what to expect, the applicants to St. Luke's pursued nursing as an alternative to other occupations.

Regardless of the expectations of average trainees, however, the apprenticeship system of work and training posed a threat to the vision of nursing leaders. Their inability to modify the image of nursing held by entrants to this field, particularly through the recruitment of higher classes of women, was only partial testament to the power of a mostly male medical establishment. Their efforts were also stalled by the majority of prospective nurses, whose enduring attitudes and beliefs embodied a very different, craft-oriented definition of nursing.

This picture is far from complete. Only the period leading up to training has been considered so far. Perhaps the expectations that the women brought to training unfairly represented what actually occurred. The next step, then, is to explore the experience of nurses' training.

4

The Limits of Duty

January 30th, Tillie and I had the afternoon off. Miss Whittaker,
superintendent of nurses, talked to us at one P.M. She accepted
us—no longer a probie but a nurse—kissed us and so forth,
thrilled!

—St. Luke's Trainee, 1929[1]

O n her first day at St. Luke's, Muriel Young, a "probie," was up with
her roommate at 6:00 A.M. She still felt tired from the previous
day's train ride to St. Paul, from her hometown of Wells, Minnesota. As instructed earlier by the superintendent of nurses, however, she
dressed in her uniform and walked the short distance from the nurses'
home to the hospital chapel by 6:30 A.M. Although the five-minute service
was over before she could focus on what was being said, she was not concerned. After all, the service was led by Reverend Pinkham, an Episcopalian, and she was a Methodist.[2]

Following chapel, Miss Young went to breakfast with the other probationers and nurses. In the midst of getting to know one another, their conversation most likely veered toward the chaos that seemed to grip the world
outside the hospital. It was 1918 and the *St. Paul Pioneer Press* was embla-
zoned with headlines of the Great War in Europe:

"ITALIANS GAIN ADVANTAGE BY SURPRISE ONSLAUGHT"
"U.S. AIRMEN VICTORS IN FIERCE HALF HOUR FIGHT"
"AMERICAN TROOPS IN FRANCE"[3]

No doubt, at least one of those present in the nurses' dining room commented on the well-publicized, urgent need for nurses in France.

On the homefront, area women were chided under the headline "MOTH-
ERS HERE LACK PATRIOTISM." The charge was that mothers were being
"negligent or indifferent in the matter of having babies and children weighed

and measured."[4] In addition, stern warnings were being made to all Minnesotans about the new party, "known as the Interallied Socialist and Labor League . . . (that) may invade the state."[5] So much unsettling news probably contributed to a "condition of lawlessness" that even touched the countryside familiar to so many of the St. Luke's trainees. A short distance from Miss Young's home, unruly crowds became such a concern that "for the first time in the history of the state military law overruled civil law," as Governor Burnquist ordered members of the First Minnesota Infantry to close all saloons in the usually sleepy town of Blooming Prairie.[6]

There was little time, though, to dwell on such matters. The immediate responsibilities of work and training could not wait. Nurses and probationers alike had to eat quickly in order to be "ready for duty" and in their assigned areas by 7:00 A.M. Miss Young eagerly awaited her duty on the first-floor ward. If she looked unusually confident as she reported to the ward, she probably explained, as she did in her application, "Four of my friends are nurses at your hospital now."[7]

On Duty

As soon as training began, the amount of time that Miss Young and the other women spent "on duty" was painstakingly recorded on their monthly record, the most important document in their files (see figures 5A–5B). On duty, the "practical" side of training, meant that a nurse was assigned to work in a part of the hospital or occasionally (during the earliest years of the program) in a private residence. Most of the nurses were on duty from their first day at St. Luke's.

Throughout the 1890s, individuals were required to spend two years, or 730 days, completing their practical training. Days spent only in classes were not credited toward meeting this total. Training school and hospital officials closely adhered to this requirement, neither exacting a large number of extra days from the nurses nor allowing them to finish early. Analysis of the women's work records revealed that they were on duty for a mean of 2.04 years, exceeding the specified number by less than fifteen days.[8] Although close accounting of days on duty remained the rule at the hospital, a dramatic change in the length of training after 1900 led to greater flexibility in the proportion of time consumed by practical training. Before considering what such flexibility in practical training meant in terms of specific numbers, however, we first need to look more closely at the larger issue of length of training.

Since 1893, nursing leaders had been working to extend the length of training to at least three years.[9] Most outspoken in this regard was Isabel

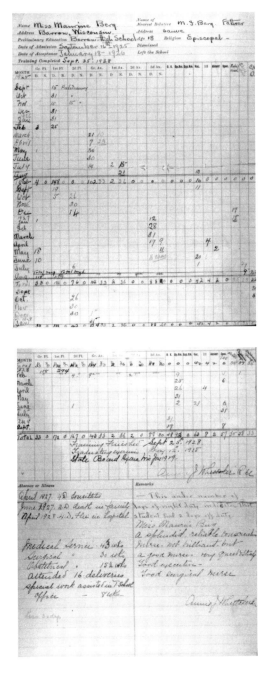

Figures 5A–5B. Monthly Record of Time on Duty, Maurine Berg, 1925–1928. From Minnesota Historical Society's Collection #152.K.20.9(B), Box 3, St. Luke's Hospital Records, St. Luke's Hospital Training School for Nurses, Folder: Maurine Berg.

Hampton, head of a prestigious training school at Johns Hopkins Hospital. Hampton had accepted leadership of the program in 1889, but only after the physician faculty agreed to accept her title of "Superintendent of Nurses and Principal of the Training School," intended to emphasize her role as an educator. Four years later, she argued for a three-year course in an address to the World Congress of Charities, Correction, and Philanthropy, held in conjunction with the Chicago World's Fair.[10]

In the hope of reforming existing nurse training into a system of academic nursing education, Hampton argued that a three-year course would permit additional instruction about theory. Her call to lengthen instruction was quickly taken up by other influential nurses, most notably Mary Adelaide Nutting, Hampton's 1894 successor at Johns Hopkins.[11] The voices of rank-and-file nurses, however, were remarkably absent from the clamor for longer training and more theory.

The balance tipped toward lengthening nursing programs due to the hospital officials, who were quick to realize the advantage that an added year of training would have for them. Ignoring the appeal of Hampton and others for a more academic model, the officials saw extended training as a way to maintain highly skilled workers, at low pay, for a longer period. Consequently, at St. Luke's and hospitals across the nation, there was little or no disagreement when the three-year proposal was considered. When brought to the attention of the St. Luke's Board of Managers in 1899, the proposal was routinely approved, effective the following year.[12]

In reflecting later on what happened, Hampton in 1905 rued the lengthening of the term of training from two to three years as it "has always been advantageous from a purely educational standpoint . . . (but) the hospital reaps the greater benefit."[13] Still, at St. Luke's the additional year was accompanied by a decrease in the proportion of total time in the program that the women spent on duty. Out of a possible total of three years, or 1095 days, the amount of time that graduates spent on duty decreased from 2.95 years from 1900 through 1910, to 2.82 years until 1923, and 2.62 years thereafter. For those who did not complete the program, time spent in training remained stable at approximately a half-year throughout the program's existence.[14]

More than anything else, the proportionate lessening of time on duty represented an easing of training requirements, since this drop was not matched by a comparable increase in academic or other expectations. Nor did the timing of this decrease, which took place on a steady basis from 1900 to 1937, correspond to particular initiatives or pressure from accrediting agencies. St. Luke's regularly reported its compliance with what had quickly become the standard for hospital programs, that is, a training period of three years or 1095 days.[15]

If, as many have argued, hospital training programs were mere expressions of an "exploitive . . . fundamentally flawed educational model," then a lessening of relative time on duty, which is what occurred at St. Luke's, is the opposite of what one would expect.[16] Of course, overall time in the program increased when vacations, absences and days devoted only to study were included in calculating days in training. Days absent, for example, ranged from zero to a full year. Yet adding these data only slightly changed the final totals. For three-year graduates, entire time in the program averaged 3.04 years for 1900 through 1910, 3.01 years for 1911 to 1923, and 2.96 years for 1924 to 1937.[17]

If exploitation existed but was not obvious from the amount of time that graduates spent on duty, then it might reasonably be expected to appear in the records of those who did not complete training. This was certainly the conclusion of an expert on early nursing education in another Midwestern state, who highlighted two incidents in which nurses had nearly completed three years of training only to be dismissed for doubtful reasons.[18] He asserted that such occurrences were common and reflected the primary importance of labor economics in the policies of training schools. Such anecdotal evidence can be misleading, however, as shown by the fact that women who failed to graduate from St. Luke's averaged only a half-year in training, throughout the life of the program. Most of these individuals actually left during their initial probationary period.[19]

Although the decreasing total days on duty cast doubt on charges of one of the most abusive practices in the hospital system of training, this does not diminish the fact that, in this system, most nursing work was done by apprentice nurses rather than graduates. As a woman who trained at St. Luke's in 1933 explained, "We (apprentice nurses) were the work horse—the hospital wouldn't have run without us."[20] During these early years of organized nursing, moreover, nurses provided virtually all hospital care, or as a trainee at the neighboring Swedish Hospital remarked, "Nursing care was hospital care."[21]

There is also little doubt that trainees faced a demanding daily schedule relative to other hospital workers. An individual's hours of duty were calculated on the basis of a seven-day-work week, with the added allowance of a "leave of absence" on one afternoon and a part of Sunday each week. Hours of duty also depended on whether a nurse was assigned to the day shift or the night shift. Until 1918, those who worked days were expected to be on duty for ten hours, with an hour's break "in the open air if the pressure of her duties and the weather permit." Thereafter, in synch with the successful demands of the larger labor movement, an eight-hour workday became the norm. On the night shift, however, hourly totals changed more slowly, from a standard of twelve hours before 1919, then ten hours through 1929, and finally eight hours.[22]

Most observers have decried the long hours on duty, as did a noted nurse historian calling it "one of the gravest problems of the profession."[23] "The preposterously long hours of service," it is reasoned, meant "educational standards did not conform even to those set for high schools."[24] Defenders of the hospital schools might have agreed that hours were long, yet insisted that it was on the job, not in the classroom, where a woman learned to be a nurse. This competing group, according to Melosh, "valued the craft skills of nursing—gentle hands, a deft injection, careful handling of the patient in pain."[25] In their minds, the cold objectivity of classroom work and an academic degree could do little to nurture the qualities of an ideal nurse. It took hours on the job to do that.

In context, the day-shift nursing schedule for apprentice nurses at St. Luke's was consistent with that of Minnesota women in manufacturing. Maximum hours per day for this group were legislated at ten in 1909. In 1914 the maximum dropped to nine.[26] It should be noted that these mandated limits did not apply to workers in sales, laundries, or textile industries. Women in those areas frequently toiled longer days than did women in hospitals or factories. Although Minnesota law did not establish a total for hours per week, the state's employers tended to follow the lead of neighboring states, where guidelines ranged from fifty-four to sixty hours per week.[27] With two half days off each week, the St. Luke's schedule fell within or below this range, hovering at sixty hours per week until 1919 and forty-eight hours per week thereafter. Still, these norms were unmistakably exceeded when the nurse regularly worked the night shift. This was true even with the two full days off that women were given after working a series of nights.

Aside from the extended time on duty, working the night shift might have been exploitive for another reason as well. The night nurse, most often a second-year apprentice or higher, frequently worked alone. Consequently, she had little opportunity to learn from either a graduate nursing supervisor or "senior nurse," as those in the last year of apprenticeship were called. Their work can be seen as minding the shop with minimal advance of education. With this in mind, it is important to pay attention to the percentage of time a woman worked on nights versus days. Such a calculation is made easy by the fact that the same meticulousness in recording total time in training was also devoted to keeping track of which shift a nurse worked. Individuals who eventually completed training spent less than 20 percent of their time working nights. Yet those who failed to complete the program—in a sense, those who must have been the most vulnerable of the trainees—worked the night shift only 7 percent of their time on duty.[28]

No doubt, the solitary work of the night nurse was a challenge far removed from the romanticized vision of the lady with the lamp peacefully making her rounds from patient to patient. However, night duty was an important part of nursing, not only inside the hospital, but also in the area where most of the trainees would ultimately find employment: the private homes of the sick. Some exposure to night duty was therefore essential to becoming a nurse. Moreover, critiques of this aspect of training have to take into account the relatively limited amount of time that individuals were assigned to night duty.

The schedule of apprentice nurses must also be seen within the context of private duty work, the main area in which most of the women would eventually seek employment. Throughout this era, a twenty-hour schedule was standard for nurses who did private duty within the hospital. Such work involved tending to a single patient while the individual was hospitalized, in essence supplementing the regular staff of apprentices and graduates. However, the nurse was paid directly by the patient, not the hospital. In many of these situations, the nurse followed her charge from the home setting, where duty often comprised a twenty-four-hour per day schedule, lasting several days at a time.[29]

Despite the rigors of private duty, it was proclaimed as early as 1890 as one of the very best fields for women: "Trained nurses receive good pay in comparison with that of the ordinary employments of women, ranging from ten dollars per week upward to twenty, thirty, or even forty dollars, according to the difficulty of the case. . . . A surgeon will sometimes refuse to take a case unless he can have the skilled nursing that he believes essential to success. . . ."[30] Still, at the urging of a group of St. Luke's graduate nurses, there was a brief discussion in 1926 of instituting a twelve-hour schedule for hospital private duty. Hospital officials summarily blocked the proposed change.[31] In contrast to private duty nurses, then, the hospital trainees faced a much less daunting schedule than the one they would likely assume after graduation, suggesting a relative lack of exploitation in the training program.

As the fleeting attempt to limit hours at St. Luke's attests, isolated groups of nurses had considerable difficulty in opposing hospital officials, most of whom had a vested interest in maintaining the status quo. This power relationship was not unique to nursing, but common within all fields. "Divided, workers were seldom a match for their employers," concluded a Minnesota labor historian in regard to employment in the first decades of the twentieth century.[32] Employers themselves were already organized into associations to protect their interests and, in particular, to eradicate unions.[33]

Yet in Minnesota and elsewhere, concerted labor organizing was increasingly challenging this status quo. In 1914, organizing among building-trades workers led to the establishment of the Hibbing Trades and Labor Assembly, a top priority of the Minnesota State Federation of Labor. In the wake of this effort, and amidst major strikes that swept the mining and timber industries in northern Minnesota, workers in St. Paul and Minneapolis also banded together. Their organizing sparked a 1917 strike against the Twin City Rapid Transit Company, opened the way for close ties between local machinists and the Socialist Party, and prompted labor's Nonpartisan League to move its headquarters from Fargo, North Dakota, to St. Paul.[34]

Twin City nurses leant support to striking workers, including helping with soup kitchens and providing first aid.[35] These workers, after all, were likely to be family, friends and neighbors. There is no evidence from this period that area nurses considered aligning with organized labor to improve their own work conditions. Nurses' support of union causes suggests that such an alliance was certainly conceivable, however.

Moreover, inroads to a partnership between nursing and labor already had been made in California. In 1913, more than a decade before the St. Luke's nurses raised the issue of hours, California became the first state to extend their "Eight-Hour Law for Women" to protect apprentice nurses. The measure was made possible with the support of ordinary nurses and a successful lobbying effort by the California Bureau of Labor. Surprisingly, perhaps, the legislation was passed over the protests of local and national leaders of nursing, as well as hospital administrators. The two most powerful organizations in nursing, the American Nurses' Association (ANA) and the National League of Nursing Education (NLNE), attacked the legislation not on its content but on the basis that it classified nursing as a trade.[36]

A major speaker at the 1915 convention of the NLNE underscored the league's concern that the California law "controls the hours of duty for nurses as it does for women in factories."[37] For nursing's elite, any link between factory workers and nurses was intolerable. The speaker concluded, "Then as speedily as possible, should we not make our training schools comply with the educational requirements of colleges and universities thus placing nursing on a professional basis?"[38] Nursing leaders also worked through the ANA to raise objections to further efforts that might bring together nursing and organized labor. In 1919, the editor of the organization's journal argued, "If the labor leaders carry out their plan for an eight-hour day, international in scope, for all workers, it would seem that the working day for this class of workers could be regulated. It would however, be more dignified if we could work it out for ourselves on a strictly professional basis."[39] The issue of dignity—a nontangible, broadly defined term—became a major point of contention between those who saw nursing as simply a good trade in a hierarchical system and those who saw nursing as a profession, not to be associated with the regimentation and subservience that characterized the industrial workforce of the time. A later piece in the ANA journal berated nurses who felt let down that the association "won't give me a job (or) won't insure an adequate income"; these were shades of trade unionism to those who relentlessly pressed for professional status. Such trade-oriented nurses were described as "skeptics (who) do not belong in a profession."[40] "Union Membership? No!" became the rallying cry of nursing leaders.[41]

These leaders exhibited faith in the potential for successful negotiation among professional partners, who it was assumed shared their goals and would therefore cooperate with nurses as peers. Overall, they overestimated the egalitarianism of medical practitioners in dealing with female-dominated occupational groups. Faced with opposition by hospital officials as well as their own leaders, it is small wonder that nurses' attempts to reduce hours of duty were easily rebuffed, such as in 1926 at St. Luke's. Yet the refusal by nursing's elite to consider any association with labor only deepened the divide between themselves and rank-and-file nurses, without bridging the divide between nurses and hospital officials.

The nurses would surely have been aware of the difference between their social standings and those of nursing's elite. Even though the notion of crossing over into a higher economic and social standing was part of working-class women's popular culture at the time, women of a higher position in the social hierarchy generally made it a point to distance themselves from those perceived as beneath them.[42] And it was these elite women in nursing who collaborated with hospital officials in determining the terms and conditions of nurses' employment. The two groups had previously been at odds over a professionalizing agenda that added a year to an already rigorous training schedule, reduced wages to apprentices, and laid the groundwork for tuition requirements. These initiatives, championed by nursing leaders promoting their vision of nursing as a profession, suited hospital officials well in terms of economic gain from each of the changes. It was a Faustian bargain that added to the burden of nurses' training and lessened the rewards of a nursing career.

Yet the overall usefulness of training to apprentice nurses was only partially a function of total hours of duty. Usefulness depended at least as much on the type of practical assignments that nurses were given—their actual clinical or work experiences. Such assignments represented "the practice essential for becoming a trained nurse." Without a thoughtful plan in making assignments, nurses' training would have been little more than drudgery, and indeed this charge was frequently heard in early nursing.

∼

Were there thoughtful plans in making assignments? "Emergencies and understaffing" dictated nurses' training, claims one observer, with the result that "the demands of the hospital for a work force meant that pupils' education was continually sacrificed to the exigencies of hospital work."[43] According to another account, "Hospital labor exigencies undoubtedly played the most important part in determining how much time a student might spend in a particular service during her three years' experience."[44] Although support for these contentions is anecdotal, the absence of published evidence to the contrary has lead to wide acceptance. However, the detailed training records of the St. Luke's nurses make it possible to look more closely and systematically at the issue of work assignments.

Like hours of duty, the type of practical work in which the women were engaged was carefully recorded, from their first assignment to their last. This information shows that most of their time was focused in two areas: medical nursing and surgical nursing (see table 4).[45] The importance of these areas was illustrated not only by their prevalence in overall percentages of work assigned to nurses, but also by the remarkable consistency over time in assigning trainees to medical and surgical wards. Across the periods, medical totals varied less than 2 percent, while surgical totals varied less than 1 percent. When the two totals are combined in each period, the percentages range from just 61.7 percent to 60.6 percent.

A consistent focus on medical and surgical nursing was prudent, considering the types of conditions for which patients sought assistance from nurses and doctors during this era. For instance, a sampling from St. Luke's "Register of the Sick" for 1914 showed that approximately a third of the patients came to the hospital with medical conditions, such as scarlet fever, an "infection of the right heel," and pyloric stenosis (narrowing of the opening between the stomach and small intestines). Slightly more came for surgical intervention, ranging from appendectomies and tonsillectomies to "the dissection of the left breast," for a fifty-six-year-old woman, and a nephrectomy (kidney removal), for a thirty-one-year-old man.[46]

Similar consistency was shown in assigning apprentice nurses to obstetrics and the nursery, the next most utilized areas in the hospital. The steady

Table 4. Practical Assignments of Graduates (in %)

	1897–1910	1911–1923	1924–1937	All
Medical	32.4	31.8	30.6	31.6
Surgical	29.3	29.2	30.0	29.5
Obstetrics and Nursery	12.6	11.8	11.7	12.0
Children	4.9	2.1	10.0	5.7
Special Nursing	4.5	2.1	0	2.1
Office Work	2.8	1.8	1.0	1.8
Floater	0	.8	1.8	.9
Diet Kitchen	5.7	7.1	4.5	5.8
Operating Room	6.2	10.1	9.6	8.7
Supplies and Dressings	1.6	3.2	.8	1.9
Number of Nurses	156	199	183	538

Source: see Table 1.

shift in maternity care from home to hospital during the early twentieth century was accompanied by the medicalization of even uncomplicated childbirth. One outcome was that women who gave birth at St. Luke's were listed as "cured," provided all went well. If problems developed for mothers or infants, three other labels might be used, depending on the results: "improved," "unimproved," or "died."[47]

The remaining areas of nursing consumed far less of the trainee's time. Work with children, although never a major emphasis of training, became more important over time, however. This is seen in the twofold percentage increase in practical assignments in this area, from the earliest years of the program to the last. Since St. Luke's never admitted a large number of children, the increase in assignments to children's care represents an effort to broaden trainees' experiences through a greater reliance on affiliated hospitals. Affiliation agreements among hospitals in a particular region had become very common by the 1920s, allowing trainees to move between institutions to gain experience not afforded in their "home" setting.

Another type of practical assignment, special nursing, is worth a closer look because it has been singled out as a glaring abuse of training. Special nursing involved sending senior apprentices—those in their last year of training—to care for private patients in their homes or in the hospital. The rationale was that "specialling" gave trainees essential preparation for private nursing. A prominent, early-twentieth-century nurse, Isabel Stewart, countered that special duty was an "unfortunate . . . bad practice . . . too obviously designed for economic rather than educational ends." She explained, "The fact is that senior students were often assigned for weeks or even months to the care of individual private patients, the fees going into the hospital treasury."[48] Stewart further asserted that from the late 1800s onward hospital programs increased rather than decreased their reliance on this practice.

Similar charges are repeated in contemporary accounts, including the following claim that hospitals sent out those in training, "as special private duty nurses and (then) confiscated the money that the students earned. . . . What resulted was a lucrative system of exploitation. A student might be kept on and on with a chronic or convalescent patient for reasons such as . . . 'the hospital wants the money,' long after any teaching value remained in the experience."[49] Still, supporters of special-duty experience had an important fact on their side—through the 1930s, private nursing remained the mainstay of most nurses after graduation. The work records from the St. Luke's nurses, moreover, reveal that special nursing never comprised a large part of training and its use steadily diminished over time, rather than increased, as Stewart argued. By 1924, in fact, this experience had disappeared from St. Luke's and was replaced with other forms of training. Still, the notion of this form of exploitation remained a standard argument for the professionalization of nursing.

Other parts of training included limited experience in the diet kitchen, where the women learned to prepare various types of meals for patients, and in the operating room, where apprentices were exposed to the growing importance of surgical intervention. The remaining practical assignments accounted for the least amount of the women's time on duty and covered a wide range of responsibilities: assisting the supervisor, most often in completing paperwork; sterilizing equipment and preparing dressings to cover wounds; and "floating," albeit figuratively not literally, to lend assistance in various areas of the hospital on an "as needed" basis. Based on the assignment records, these additional responsibilities only supplemented an apprentice's practice. Most of the women's time remained set aside for work that regularly brought them into contact with patients in the most common areas of nursing.

The consistency of the apprentices' practical assignments at St. Luke's seems to defy at least some of the arguments that the training system abused its trainees. This is particularly true when the pattern of assignments is seen within the context of a forty-year span that included fifteen different superintendents of nursing, nine different hospital superintendents, and fluctuating patient admissions to more than a dozen hospital wards.[50] Indeed, the regularity of assignments at St. Luke's would be difficult to match in contemporary, university-based nursing programs, where the primary aim is clearly understood as education rather than service. It is even more remarkable, then, to find such regularity in an unremarkable early-twentieth-century hospital program, where service and education were closely intertwined.

If "emergencies and understaffing" dictated nurses' training, would there not appear a less uniform pattern of practical assignments—one whose changes in training patterns would coincide with frequent changes in patient admissions and staffing? These records reveal one training program where training was on a par with service. In view of this evidence, other records at other institutions should be explored to further test the accepted thinking that early training was essentially a system of exploitation.

The exploitation theory also posits that apprentices had scant opportunity to learn from more experienced nurses, a claim that once again sees nursing programs relegated to little more than instruments of staffing for hospitals. Clearly, programs would have suffered from having too few graduate nurses available to assist in training. At St. Luke's, a full-time instructor was not even listed in accreditation reports until 1918, and even then her title included both general supervisor and instructor, which looks bad for the formal learning experience of trainees.[51] From the standpoint of the academic ideal to which nursing leaders aspired, nursing education could have seemed almost nonexistent in hospital programs such as St. Luke's at the turn of the century, with slow progress thereafter.

There is, however, another facet of this issue: the definition of instructor. Was this a separate job category or simply part of the obligation owed by more seasoned workers to mentor the more junior workers? At St. Luke's and elsewhere, all of those who supervised trainees were considered to be instructors, even though formal instruction generally comprised only part of their responsibilities. Though an opportune view for the hospital, it is also consistent with craft traditions, according to which skills are learned on the job, from experienced artisans. In contemporary trades, new apprentices learn not only from master craftsmen, but from journeymen and others with more experience than themselves.

The 1901 training school bulletin for St. Luke's acknowledged four experienced nurses as instructors: the superintendent of nursing, the superintendent of the hospital, and two head nurses.[52] These four graduate nurses supervised a total of thirty-four apprentices. Of this number, fifteen were senior nurses, or those nearing completion of training. Those who had reached this level, not unlike journeymen, were expected to add their experience and skill in training "junior nurses." This craft-linked tradition of teaching and learning continued, but by 1911 the training program boasted five supervisors, who now also functioned as members of the "teaching staff." This number increased to twelve, in 1921, and to thirteen by the last decade of the program.[53]

Careful consideration of the issue of teaching suggests a craft-based way of viewing the form taken by hospital training. For the women of St. Luke's, training was as important as service, at least from the standpoint of their length of training, hours of duty, and practical assignments. However, these findings do not explain how academic instruction was handled within the program or, more fundamentally, how the women conceived of this part of their work.

REPORTS, REALITY, AND THEORY

Practical assignments were being meticulously recorded at St. Luke's two years before the first reference was made to the nurses' "theoretical work," as academic instruction was called. In 1899, six courses were listed for nurses: gynecological nursing, obstetrics, "nervous and insane," orthopedics, children's diseases, and eye and ear. Initially, all of the courses were taught by physicians. Within three years, however, the number of courses had doubled and teaching responsibilities shifted increasingly to nurses.[54]

Other courses were added periodically. These included a lecture series on "skin and venereal diseases," sanitation, "operating room technic [sic]," emergency and first aid, and massage. Then, in 1930, St. Luke's initiated one of the most consequential changes in terms of the nurses' academic work. The training program began requiring women to complete a semester of preliminary coursework at the University of Minnesota, prior to entering the hospital. Required studies included basic sciences and the history of nursing.

Most of these developments would have cheered nursing leaders, as they continued to press for their vision of professional nursing. They would have been especially pleased, had they known, to see that the increase in courses at St. Luke's was documented in regular reports to two accreditation agencies, the Boards of Nurse Examiners in both Minnesota and New York. Dual accreditation was intended to assure respect for the program both locally and nationally, in addition to guaranteeing that graduates would be eligible for registration in both states.

Registration was a reform supported not only by the nursing elite, but also by rank-and-file nurses who saw it as a way to protect their livelihood.[55] As established by various state nurse-practice acts, registration gave graduate nurses from accredited schools the right to the title, "registered nurse," while claims to the label "nurse" remained unfettered. United by "this common cause," explained a St. Paul nurse, nurses were "vibrating with a single interest."[56] Following a statewide campaign aimed at influencing lawmakers, Minnesota's nurse practice act "passed with little difficulty" and was signed by Gov. Albert Johnson in April 1907.[57] A three-year waiver period meant the act actually took effect in 1910. At approximately the same time, the graduate nurse association in St. Paul, which controlled entry into private duty within the city, voted to make state registration one of its qualifications for membership.[58]

As news spread about the passage of the nurse practice act, "hospitals all over the state," including St. Luke's, "were writing to learn what they could do to qualify."[59] They were understandably concerned about remaining competitive in attracting trainees and in guaranteeing positions for their graduates. What hospital officials learned is that their program would need to be accredited by the newly formed Minnesota Board of Nurse Examiners. At the earliest opportunity, then, St. Luke's joined other hospitals in the state in seeking accreditation.[60]

The move toward registration and accreditation, like the introduction of formal coursework, seemed to reinforce the notion that nursing was on a clear path toward a solidly professional future. Yet closer scrutiny reveals serious problems with this idea at St. Luke's. To start with, the extent to which theory was emphasized at St. Luke's was not measured as systematically as the practical work. Documentation of academic work, in contrast to practice, was erratic and often contradictory. For instance, the "number of lessons" that apprentices covered in a course, and thus the amount of time they devoted to a particular subject, was not recorded until 1912.[61] Even after that time, the number of class hours was frequently omitted from individual records or, when included, often conflicted with totals provided for other apprentices.

Course grades, like the number of class hours, were often missing. Even when assigned, grades had little significance. Officially, the program maintained a failing level that ranged from 50 percent to 75 percent. Yet nurses frequently continued their training with "ratings," as grades were also called, below this range. Nor was any record kept of whether an individual attended classes.[62] Such practices were difficult to reconcile with the more visible symbols of an increasing emphasis on academics. Further consideration of the accreditation process, however, helped in sorting out this puzzle.

Accreditation largely depended on voluntary self-reporting from the training program. The New York Board, in particular, relied exclusively on such reporting.[63] Thus, between 1909 and 1939 the superintendents of the training school dutifully filed yearly reports with this board. Each could be confident that her assessment would go unchallenged, because the only attempt to confirm what she wrote was the stipulation that the "presiding officer" of the hospital would cosign the report. As previously noted, the presiding officer or superintendent of the hospital shared overlapping responsibilities with the superintendent of the training program. It was hardly an effective system of verification.

Not surprisingly, then, the superintendents' accrediting reports specified exactly the same courses as those required by the accrediting body. The superintendent was even less forthcoming in mentioning any of the widespread irregularities evident in the academic records of the apprentices. Clearly they would have understood, however, that the lack of a uniform grading standard and the failure to keep track of class hours or the number of courses that trainees attended meant that the most basic expectations of the New York Board were not being met. The situation was only slightly different with the local board.

St. Luke's was accredited by the Minnesota Board for the entire thirty years it was eligible, from 1907 to 1937. What this generally entailed was that the superintendent of either the hospital or nursing simply completed the necessary forms and submitted them without further question.[64]

The board conducted only four "surveys" or on-site inspections.[65] After its first inspection, in 1920, the board concluded that "St. Luke's T.S. (training school) is . . . one of the best." Surveyors emphasized: "With the exception of the utuility [*sic*] rooms which were not very tidy and showed need of supervision the rooms and corridors were clean and orderly. There is a social director here in charge of the nurses' home and the home is apparently kept in good condition."[66] Only after making these points did the surveyors note: "Faculty and class schedule all made up."[67] There was no mention of what this schedule involved or the extent to which it was being implemented. Also missing were any comments about irregularities involving grades, attendance, or amount of time spent in class. Instead of theory, the focus was decidedly on physical aspects of hospital training and practice, defusing the very academic thrust that had propelled the accreditation drive.

Subsequent inspections involved a similar approach. Among the most important recommendations were:

- If possible, each floor be supplied with a sterilizer for bedpans and basins.
- Regular conferences. Rounds to be made with a notebook . . . each supervisor sometime during the twenty-four hours after the conference to call all her nurses together and to give them the notes.
- Yale locks to be put on medicine closets. Narcotics to be kept in separate place.
- That, when infectious cases are isolated, strict contagious tech-

nique be used to give . . . the benefit of such practice.
· Recommended ice cap covers.[68]

As in the initial inspection in 1920, later visits highlighted material considerations aimed more at practice than classroom study. In particular, the recommendation about "rounds"—the supervisor's regular review of a nurse's work with each patient—was intended to benefit training by strengthening oversight of apprentices. Likewise, the suggestion involving "infectious cases" was aimed at providing trainees with sufficient opportunity to practice strict contagious technique. Such technique included detailed methods of adorning protective clothing and of handling the patient and hospital equipment. As before, issues related to classroom education were not raised.[69]

The lack of attention to academics in the survey recommendations, along with the disregard for the reality of classroom learning evident in the self-reports, suggests that the symbols of an increasing emphasis on theory were just that, purely symbols. By listing expanded course offerings and seeking accreditation, St. Luke's seemed to be rallying behind the efforts of nursing leaders. In truth, however, the day-to-day experience of apprentice nurses was relatively unchanged by these occasional brushes with academics. For them, nursing remained "impossible to learn . . . from any book," as Nightingale had stressed decades before.[70] Instead, for the women of St. Luke's and thousands of other trainees, "practical manual nursing . . . (could) only be thoroughly learnt in the wards of a hospital," adding to the confusion about nursing's apparent dual status as a craft and a profession.[71]

A shift in emphasis was evident, however, in the final survey by the Minnesota Board. Following the visit in 1934, surveyors made three recommendations, all of which focused on theory. These included enlarging "the Nursing School Committee . . . to include an educator," organizing "a program of teaching in the classroom with appropriate and progressive rotation of service," and appointing "an additional person qualified for the position of Director of the School."[72] In a follow-up letter board members explained that these recommendations were taken from the "Grading Committee Reports," the culmination of a nursing education reform effort sponsored by the leaders of the American Nurses' Association, the National Organization for Public Health Nursing, and the National League of Nursing Education.[73] Given this sponsorship, the conclusion by Isabel Stewart that the reports "agreed with . . . the observations and criticisms of leaders in the nursing field covering a period of many years" was less than startling.[74]

With some sense of how their comments would be regarded by St. Luke's, the members of the Minnesota Board encouraged hospital and training school officials to "at least scan the reports" of the Grading Committee. Miss Grace Scott, who at the time had assumed the dual role of nursing and hospital superintendent, seemed to pay little attention to the board's recommendations or the Grading Committee Reports. Nor did others involved with the program. None of the board's recommendations were implemented, except to change the title of "instructor" to "director."[75]

One has to wonder if the Minnesota Board's tone reflected an acknowledgment of the practical recalcitrance of St. Luke's and training programs toward professionalization. The Minnesota Board of Nurse Examiners, which represented nursing's elite in Minnesota, had moved toward a more academic view of nursing, as espoused by national leaders. Yet St. Luke's resisted any change from its apprenticeship system. Instead, strong academic recommendations based on the 1934 survey prompted newly hired officials, hospital superintendent Miss Jean Campbell and nursing superintendent Miss Myrtle Paulson, to reevaluate the hospital's need for a training school. They concluded, along with a majority of the hospital board, that it would be nearly as economical to hire more graduate nurses to staff the hospital than to rely on the current mixture of graduates and students.[76] Consequently, in 1935, St. Luke's stopped admitting prospective nurses. The training school closed just two years later.

There was no coincidence in the ending of the long relationship between the hospital and the nursing program so soon after the 1934 survey. Close inspection of the nurses' academic records reveals scant interest in classroom matters, something that had not been problematic even under accreditation review, until the 1934 questions by the Minnesota Board. In contrast, the nurses' practical assignments showed that program officials never wavered from their commitment to a carefully planned, consistent schedule of practical work and training. Of course, the deepening depression and the related decrease in private-duty nursing jobs helped to lure more graduate nurses to the hospital staff. Still, St. Luke's was not forced to take this path. The training school was in no danger of being closed by the Minnesota Board and the 1934 recommendations could have been implemented with little time and expense.

Despite having endured previous economic downturns, two wars, and devastating episodes of disease, none at the St. Luke's school appeared ready for the required change in direction implicit in the 1934 survey. This seemingly sudden shift to a more academic focus did not fit the image of nursing that seemed to underlie the approach to training in effect for more than three decades. One might argue that a change in view may have been occurring for some time among the nurses, but would not have been revealed by the academic and practical records just discussed. Thus it could

be argued that the demise of the program resulted more from the preferences of the two new hospital officials. Miss Campbell and Miss Paulson
might have preferred to run the hospital more independently than functioning as links in an increasingly professionalized, externally influenced,
chain of command. Rather than demonstrating widespread resistance to
change, the decision to close St. Luke's might have been consistent with
their interpretation of the nature of nursing. The next step, then, is to
explore what nursing meant to the women of St. Luke's during training, as
expressed in their own words.

5

Laying Claim to Caring

November 19th, 1928: First snowfall. The first time I gave a bed bath. Gave one to Mr. Van Camp—a young flirt. I told him to finish the bath and he said he didn't need to. The sap. Complimented me to Miss Alson.

—St. Luke's Trainee, 1928[1]

ontemporary nursing leaders have rallied around the idea of caring, claiming this as the core of nursing practice and thus the field's "special knowledge." Consistent with professionalization theory, identifying, developing, and successfully laying claim to special knowledge is viewed as crucial to establishing nursing as a full-fledged profession.[2] As elaborated in a frequently cited article in nursing, a profession is "distinguished by a domain of inquiry that represents a shared belief among it members regarding its reason for being."[3] Moreover, two prominent nurses assert, "It is the common link to caring that brings nurses together."[4] Another leader adds, "Caring is the central, dominant and unifying feature of nursing."[5] The titles of well-known, contemporary works in nursing highlight the claim to caring: *Nursing as Caring; Care: The Essence of Nursing and Health; The Primacy of Caring;* and *Nursing: The Philosophy and Science of Caring.*[6]

The argument for caring is generally legitimized by asserting its historic basis. This argument typically proceeds as follows: "Care forms the basic core of nursing actions. Traditionally nurses have described the act of administering to patients as care behaviors."[7] Yet the nurses upon whom this view is based are frequently omitted from such descriptions. In other words, caring as the essence of nursing is assumed. When nurses from the past are cited, they tend to be from the professional elite. For example, the words of Isabel Stewart underpin a warning in the *Journal of Professional Nursing* that "caring is slowly disappearing" from nursing. Stewart is quoted as insisting: "The real essence of nursing . . . lies not in the mechanical details of execution, not yet in the dexterity of the performer, but in the creative imagination, the sensitive spirit, and the intelligent understanding lying back of these techniques and skills. Without these, nursing may become a highly skilled trade, but it cannot be a profession."[8]

Even in those accounts that draw on information from rank-and-file nurses, the assumption of caring is imposed on historical subjects rather than discovered in their records. In one of the best-known works on nursing history, the conclusion that nurses were "ordered to care" is reached without really questioning the underlying premise that equates nursing and caring.[9] However, when we first suggested examining this premise, we were chided by one nurse historian who remarked that we could not possibly be questioning the relationship between nursing and caring. She added, "I infer that what (actually) intrigues you . . . (is) to spell out and verify the conflicts and tensions (around) . . . being a caring nurse."[10] For her, the two terms were synonymous. Another nursing scholar acknowledged our intent accurately but insisted that to understand nursing and caring we would have to "go back to the original source—Nightingale," rather than relying on the statements of ordinary nurses.[11] In the field of intellectual history such an argument might be normative but a social history such as this study relies precisely on just that—the experiences of ordinary nurses, as best they can be recreated from extant records.

In current discussions, the claim to caring is frequently linked to feminist ideas put forward in the theoretical debates of the1980s that placed women at center stage instead of in the periphery of society. As a well-known nursing author explains in the *American Journal of Nursing,* "women's caring work," nursing, must be esteemed by society if we are to "move away from the masculine dream toward a new feminine future."[12] The fact that society "systematically undervalues care," according to another account, is the primary reason for nursing's difficulty in becoming "a woman-valued work group."[13]

This construct ignores the negative consequences for women of being seen as "natural" caregivers, such as their economic dependence on men and their low status in the hierarchy of paid work.[14] Glazer, a sociologist, clarifies the gender divide that tends to frame such discussions of caring: the "view of the relative passivity of women finds a complement in feminist views of women as more cooperative and relational, more caring and less aggressive than men and . . . less mechanistic and hierarchical."[15] In this way caring, linked to specifically female historical actors, is correlated with psychological attributes of passivity and even submissiveness. "The 'feminine' principles," emphasizes a feminist scholar, "correspond to the historical roots of nursing—caring, nurturance, receptivity."[16]

Yet, as one critic challenges, "if caring is really the 'essence of nursing' then it must be demonstrated and not simply proclaimed."[17] It must also be defined. This leads to the fundamental question: How solid is the historical relationship between caring and nursing, before more recent turns to a psychological definition of caring? Among the women engaged in the day-to-day work of nursing in the early twentieth century, was their work seen as caring, or closely related to caring? If not, how did these individuals conceive of their field?[18]

~

In searching for a deeper understanding of what nursing meant to the women of St. Luke's, it is important to keep in mind that once beyond probation, a trainee was thereafter referred to as "nurse." Terms such as "student" or "pupil" were conspicuously absent from hospital dialogue and written records. So no longer a "probie," Verdel Iverson, a young woman who came to St. Luke's in 1925, from Radcliffe, Iowa, was described during the remainder of her first year as "a good strong nurse."[19] This was according to Maple Baer, a charge nurse and a 1922 graduate of the hospital.

In her second year, the woman was characterized as "a reliable and conscientious nurse" by Elmyra Nelson, the assistant night supervisor and a 1925 graduate of St. Luke's. Soon after, another supervisor observed, "The patients all liked Miss Iverson very much. She is a very good nurse." In her final year of training, a charge nurse explained that Miss Iverson was "a very capable nurse and pleasant to work with." The superintendent of training offered her own terse summary, "Good Nurse in Practical Work." In total, seven different graduate nurses provided written evaluations of this individual during her work and training. Each one referred to her as a nurse.[20]

There was equal certainty during training about just which qualities a woman must possess to earn the title of nurse. Moreover, these were the same qualities that had been emphasized earlier during the application process. Above all, a nurse had to have physical strength and endurance, common sense, and a strong personality. A nurse was accordingly criticized in 1925 for having "neither a strong physique nor personality." Gusta Erstad, the immediate supervisor, added "she lacks self-reliance." The superintendent of nursing endorsed this opinion, stating there is "not much force to her."[21]

Others, such as Marie Weisbecker, merited praise from their supervisors for demonstrating the attributes of a nurse. For instance, the charge nurse in the operating room commended Miss Weisbecker for being "very neat and (having) confidence in her own ability." Her obstetrical supervisor

handled, managed, controlled

said, "Miss Weisbecker showed good judgment with patients while on the floor." In addition, the assistant superintendent of nursing pointed out, she has "splendid health and excellent common sense."[22]

These qualities, and the authority that came with being called a nurse, were integral to an overall definition that infused all aspects of nursing at St. Luke's. A crucial part of this definition was repeated when Evelyn Ferrell, similar to many trainees before and after her, was praised in 1923 as "a good adaptable all around nurse" based on her "way of handling patients."[23] Indeed, "handling patients" was the most frequently used phrase to describe nursing at St. Luke's. Among the last group of women to train at the hospital, one was portrayed as "a large girl—strong and capable in handling patients," and another as "very capable in manual handling of patients."[24]

The way in which a nurse handled patients could be a source of criticism as well as praise. For instance, a superintendent of nurses wrote to an older sister of a trainee, decrying the younger woman's "practical nursing." The main problem, the superintendent explained, was that "your sister . . . find(s) it difficult to handle patients." She added the following advice, "(your sister) tells me that she is very much interested in English with library training, and to be very candid with you, I feel she would be more successful in this line than in nursing."[25]

Only slightly less often than handling, nurses were judged in terms of how they "controlled" and "managed" patients. A "ward report" from 1929, for example, described Alice Dahl as a nurse whose "patients were always well under control."[26] Another woman was commended in 1933 because "she is interested in work (and) manages patients well."[27] Still other nurses received similar approval for having "managed children well" and for having "good control of babies."[28] At St. Luke's, nurses could hardly ask for higher compliments than these.

Discussions with several women who trained and worked at St. Luke's, most of whom were in their eighties when interviewed, helped to explain what was involved in handling, controlling, or managing patients. Sitting on the edge of her bed in a St. Paul–area nursing home, Edythe Newman, a 1936 graduate, remarked, "I don't think I'd like the nursing nowadays— it's the aides and the practical nurses who really deal with patients." She continued, "in those days a patient was a patient and they stayed in bed and you did everything *for* (emphasis original) them. You gave them their bath and brought them the bed pan. . . ."[29] Nursing in this description, "deal(ing) with patients," meant taking an active role in doing things for people, particularly carrying out procedures.

Miss Newman was not alone in her thinking. Toward the end of September 1928, a young woman named Grace Bakke eagerly looked up at the stone columns that framed the entrance to St. Luke's and bravely climbed the steps to the hospital to begin her work as a nurse. She had just arrived from the small, close-knit, central-Minnesota farming community of Granite Falls, and the city surrounding St. Luke's appeared menacing. St. Paul was in the midst of a prohibition-related crime wave, with prostitution, gambling, and dozens of speakeasies flourishing just blocks away from the hospital. Violence was common, with two men and a woman shot down near the state capitol in what local newspapers called "the third outbreak of gang warfare in the Twin Cities within two weeks."[30] Yet Miss Bakke's determination to be a nurse never wavered as she resolutely took on the task of recording her daily observations of her new vocation in several tersely worded diaries. She emphasized her first experiences involving procedures and patients, such as the story quoted at the beginning of this chapter about Miss Bakke giving her first bed bath.[31] Miss Bakke made similar comments about "the first time I gave a bed pan"; the first "evening toilet—made sure they (patients) brushed their teeth and (I) gave back rubs"; and the first enema she gave. On May 4, 1929, she proclaimed, "Shot my first hypo!" With equal excitement she also noted the day "I received my first paycheck—on fourth floor."[32]

Another nurse, originally from St. Paul's Westside, kept a scrapbook that covered her years at St. Luke's, 1929 to 1932. On one page was a poem that she read aloud, saying that it described her experience with a patient while on night duty:

> The patient grows better night by night,
> Because some nurse in her evening plight
> Forces the fluids and forces them strong
> Keeps on forcing them all night long
> She makes drinks from oranges, from lemons, from grapes
> And Oh, what a lot of fruits it takes,
> She forces the fluid in great many ways
> By temperature sponges, hot packs and on Trays. . . . [33]

In this example, and the others presented above, the meaning of nursing is clear. Nursing meant taking the lead, assuming an assertive, vigorous role in carrying out common and not-so-common procedures, including bathing a patient and forcing fluids. Nursing also meant being paid for one's work, even while in training. Consistent with Miss Bakke, this last individual set aside an entire page of her scrapbook to display "My last pay envelop."

Recognizing a similar need for qualities of strength and forcefulness in nursing, the author of a turn-of-the-century guide to nursing highlighted the following lines from the poet Wordsworth:

A traveler betwixt life and death;
The reason firm, the temperate will,
Endurance, foresight, strength, and skill;
A perfect woman, nobly plann'd,
To warn, to comfort, and command. . . . [34]

The ability to warn, comfort, and command, beyond its poetic sound, is not so distant from the St. Luke's nurses' own description of handling, managing, and controlling. Moreover, the strength that underlay all of these designations was central to everyday nursing practice.

The day-to-day routine of nursing was illustrated in the case records, or descriptions of work with specific patients, that were kept by the nurses. Two examples are included below, the first from the day shift and the second from the night shift. Both focus on patients on medical units, with undiagnosed illnesses. The nurse's work with one particular patient during the day unfolded as follows:

7:15–7:30 A.M.	Feeding patient.
7:30–8:00 A.M.	Medications (given); patient toileted.
8:00–8:30 A.M.	Patient bathed; alcohol rub; linen changed.
9:30–10:00 A.M.	Application of splint.
10:20–10:30 A.M.	Oral hygiene.
11:20–11:30 A.M.	Temperature taken.
12:20–12:45 P.M.	Feeding patient.
12:55–1:00 P.M.	Medications (given); patient toileted; patient prepared for rest.[35]

In addition to this patient, the nurse in this situation was responsible for two other patients during the same period.

With the exception of the application of a splint, the description from the day shift included regularly performed tasks. In contrast, the night nurse found herself in a situation in which she had to concentrate on changes in the patient's condition. Her work proceeded as follows:

8:45 P.M.	Vital signs taken. (Patient) complains of headache. Patient seems very excitable. Talks and laughs a great deal. Ice cap to head.
10:10 P.M.	Patient very noisy. Complains of hand feeling numb. Acts drowsy.
10:40 P.M.	(Patient) taken to Physiotherapy Room II. Drank 2 cups

of water. Had difficulty in getting into bed. Patient complains of being cold. Extreme heat applied. Patient per-
spiring.

11:00 P.M.   Patient quiet and appears to be sleeping.[36]

As the night nurse's experience shows, nursing was not just a matter of
carrying out fixed procedures, but varied depending on a patient's condition. Considered together, the different examples also underscore the
forceful, physical, and pragmatic actions that were required of a nurse if
she was to effectively handle patients. Her actions were all the more important during an era that preceded many of today's commonly used medical
treatments, such as the administration of antibiotics—an era in which the
main offering of hospitals was, unquestionably, nursing skill.

Yet nursing entailed more than simply handling patients. In 1920, for
instance, a senior nursing apprentice named Gertrude Rothschild was
hailed as "a very capable charge nurse" for being able to "manage both
patient and doctors."[37] This praise is noteworthy because it contradicts
usual arguments that apprenticeship stressed passivity and subservience. It
was through the apprenticeship system, according to such arguments, that
"the rank and file in nursing were persuaded to believe in their inferior-
ity."[38] If true, however, such a system would have left few if any individuals
who were able to manage doctors, let alone patients.

Miss Rothschild's praise is also one of the few references to physicians in
the records of the St. Luke's nurses. This was unexpected, given the deeply
entrenched notion that "loyalty and deference to the physician . . . were
stressed" in hospital programs.[39] Certainly one outcome of this stress would
have been that physicians were mentioned with some regularity, at the very
least in regard to disciplinary issues which, as discussed in the next chapter,
were described in meticulous detail. If there was a near absence of comments
regarding doctors, however, the records were replete with descriptions of
how nurses managed "the help," primarily maids and male attendants, and
"junior nurses," those individuals who were relatively new to training.[40] In
one example, a senior apprentice was criticized by the superintendent of
nursing because "she seemed to antagonize many of the junior nurses." As a
result, "Her associates . . . did not enjoy working under her."[41]

The reality of work and practice at St. Luke's was that the world of the
nurse and the world of the physician were widely separated. Of necessity,
the two worlds occasionally converged, but as swiftly as they came together
they once again parted. According to Baer, a well-known nurse historian,
the reason "this separateness of practice area . . . has never been, substantially recognized . . . (is) because medicine and nursing share a locus of

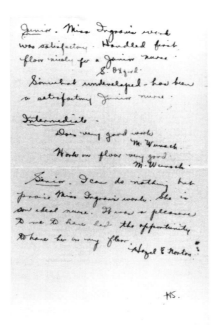

Figures 6A–6B. Efficiency Record, Florence Ingram, 1925. From Minnesota Historical Society's Collection #152.K.20.8(F), Box 2, St. Luke's Hospital Records, St. Luke's Hospital Training School for Nurses, Folder: Florence K. Ingram.

work, a clientele group, and have certain overlapping functions." Consequently, "this notion of relative amounts of authority is seen as the issue when it is not the issue."[42]

The issue, as Nightingale and subsequent nurses argued, was that women had to be in charge of women because "in disciplinary matters a woman only can understand a woman."[43] Even the insistence on obedience to doctors, according to one historian, is best interpreted as "a shrewd understanding of the problems of women exercising control in a male dominated society."[44] What existed was an unwritten, but commonly understood trade-off, according to which "nurses would obey doctors' medical orders but those doctors had no rights to direct nursing work or to discipline an individual nurse."[45]

Aside from handling patients and managing attendants, maids, and junior nurses, the nurse was also expected to oversee the physical setting in which she worked. Consequently, a nurse was immediately applauded if she "manage(d) the sick room well," "left the ward in good condition," or "handled (the) floor nicely" (see figures 6A–6B).[46] Yet just as quickly, she was criticized for the opposite actions, such as a 1928 nurse who was chided for leaving "the floor in a mess."[47] If a nurse excelled in the daunting task of handling patients, workers, and ward, she earned the ultimate praise, "an all around good nurse," as Elmyra Nelson did in 1922.[48] Before earning this accolade, however, her ability to handle such disparate responsibilities would have been judged against the overall goal of nursing.

~

At St. Luke's the goal of nursing consistently focused on a tangible outcome. This was similar to artisans in other fields, such as seamstresses and shoemakers. Handling and managing were intended to produce, in the words of the nurses, "work that has a finished appearance."[49] This phrase, more than any other, was used to gauge an individual's overall success in nursing.

Alice Thompson was judged to be a "conscientious nurse," for example, because "her work presented a finished appearance and her patients were fond of her."[50] Several years later, a Wisconsin nurse was deemed to be "a splendid worker," based on the fact that "her work always looks finished . . . her ward is in good condition at all times."[51] With the same goal in mind, supervisors praised one of the last women to graduate from St. Luke's for doing "neat, finished bedside nursing."[52] Conversely, another nurse was admonished because "she is a slow worker and her work does not present a finished appearance."[53]

Like the actions of handling, managing, and controlling, the goal of finished work encompassed more than a first glance might suggest. Beyond simply completing or finishing a task, it referred to the more general and observable end result of nursing work. Of course, specific results tended to vary depending on the situation. In the diet kitchen, for instance, finished work was equated with "serv(ing) lovely trays" and "taking an interest in having the trays look nice," whereas finished work in the operating room meant "keeping equipment in order and ... good condition."[54] In the broadest range of nursing situations, finished work was demonstrated by maintaining "tidy rooms" and a "neat ward (or floor)."[55] Indeed, one of the earliest and most repeated instructions that each nurse received was that the "appearance of (the) ward should have a finished look at 7 A.M. (and) ... at 7 P.M."[56]

Nurses were evaluated in regard to their direct involvement with patients in similarly concrete terms. "Keeping babies clean and dry," for example, constituted "neat, finished appearing work" for an individual assigned to the nursery.[57] In general, a nurse's bedside work was measured on the basis of whether or not patients were properly positioned, in orderly surroundings, and that "routine work ... was thoroughly completed."[58] The latter included such tasks as feeding, bathing, and "toileting" patients. Finished work with patients also required that additional "procedures were properly done," including techniques and treatments that went well beyond the routine.[59] If a nurse's work with patients presented a finished appearance in all of these aspects, then patients would "speak well of the nurse," or so it was assumed (see figures 7 and 8).[60]

Whether the work was routine or not, it generally required a nurse to follow specific and detailed steps. To make a finished-appearing bed at St. Luke's, for example, a nurse had to first assemble eleven pieces of "equipment" before proceeding through the twelve steps of bed making. This was a simple matter, however, compared to the eighteen steps for administering a hot pack or the twenty-one steps necessary for giving a bath. Yet all of these were routine tasks, overshadowed by the even greater detail and skill demanded in more complex procedures, such as urinary catheterization, dressing burns, gastrogavage (feeding the patient through a tube to the stomach), and hypodermoclysis (injection of fluids into subcutaneous tissue).[61]

Meticulous attention to detail was the norm not only at St. Luke's, but elsewhere as well. In one study of nurses' work from 1920 to 1939, the author described the elaborate procedure involved in administering a hypodermic injection. To prepare for this procedure, the nurse began by setting up "a small tray with the medication, a sterile jar with alcohol and sterile sponges, one jar containing the needles, another with the alcohol and hypodermic syringe, a small bottle of alcohol and one of sterile water, an alcohol lamp and spoon, and matches." In its entirety, the process of

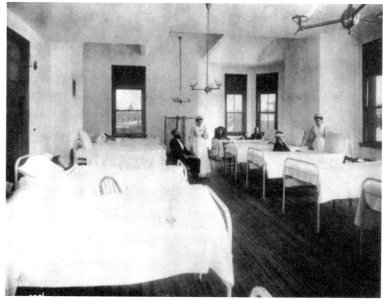

Figure 7. Finished-Appearing Patients, Workers, and Ward, ca. 1900. From Minnesota Historical Society's Collection #143.B.20.4(B), Box 8, United Hospital Records, Folder: Interior views, old hospital, 1897–1930.

doing finished-appearing work in giving an injection demanded that a nurse carefully implement no less than seventeen steps:

1. Have medication ready.
2. Test your needle.
3. Place needle with stilette in spoon and cover with water.
4. Boil over lamp two minutes.
5. Place cover over wick.
6. Rinse out barrel of syringe.
7. Draw amount of water required into syringe.
8. Discard water remaining in spoon.
9. Attach needle to syringe and remove stilette.
10. Place tablets on spoon and dissolve with water in syringe.
11. Draw prepared fluid into syringe, taking up last drop.
12. Expel air from syringe.
13. Pick up sponge on point of needle and replace tray in cupboard.
14. Cleanse the area, make a cushion of flesh and insert quickly.
15. Withdraw slightly and insert fluid slowly.
16. Withdraw needle quickly, massage area gently with a circular motion.

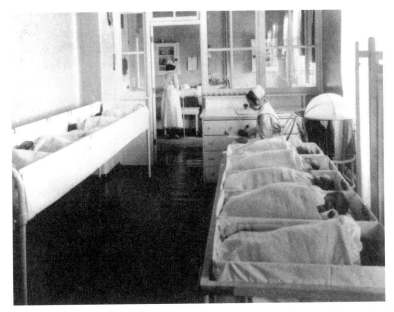

Figure 8. Finished-Appearing Nursery, 1910. From Minnesota Historical Society's Collection #143.B.20.4(B), Box 8, United Hospital Records, Folder: Interior views, old hospital, 1897-1930.

> 17. Chart time, medication and initials immediately after giving drug, and mark off in order book.[62]

The ability to produce neat, finished-appearing work, by mastering hypodermic injections and the many other complex tasks of nursing, must have seemed a daunting undertaking for new entrants to the hospital program. Of course, the need to flawlessly execute the intricacies of nursing work also provided the justification for the months and years of practice to which each woman committed herself. Yet practice alone was of little value unless the nurse could also command the physical strength and skill that underlay nearly all of the procedures that she was called upon to do. If successful in mustering these qualities and completing a particular procedure, the nurse's expertise was duly noted on the "Record of Nursing Procedures" (see figures 9A–9B). This record was second in importance only to the monthly record, which documented time in training. For all of the women, it was consistently used to track their progress, with the title of graduate nurse limited to apprentices who demonstrated finished-appearing procedures in class and actual clinical situations.

The central importance of carrying out procedures epitomized nursing's

ST. LUKE'S HOSPITAL
TRAINING SCHOOL FOR NURSES

Record of Nursing Procedures

NAME Ponsness, Louise CLASS 1928

	DEMONSTRATION		FLOORS		
	Class	Pupil	1	2	3
Care of Room or Ward	XX	XX	X	X	X
Care of Service Room, Bath, Toilet	XX	XX	X	X	X
Care of Linen Room	XX	XX	X	X	X
Admission and Discharge of Patient	XX	XX	X		
Feeding of Helpless Patients	XX	XX	X	X	X
Care of Bed and Bedding	XX	XX	X	X	X
Bed Making with Patient	XX	XX	X	X	X
Bed Making—Ambulance Bed	XX	XX	X	X	
Ether Bed	XX	XX	X	X	
Fracture Bed	XX	XX			
Up Patient's Bed	XX	XX	X	X	X
Preparation for and assisting with Tub Bath	XX	XX	X		
Bed Bath	XX	XX	X	X	X
Evening Toilet	XX	XX	X	X	X
Moving and Lifting Patients—In Bed	XX	XX	X	X	X
To Chair	XX	XX	X	X	
To Stretcher	XX	XX		X	
Use of Pillows, Pads, Air-Cushions	XX	XX	X	X	X
Use of Back Rest, Cradles	XX	XX	X	X	
Preparation for the night	XX	XX	X	X	X
Special Care of Back, Mouth, Teeth	XX	XX	X		
Washing the Hair	XX	XX			
Care of Infected Hair	XX	XX			
Preparation for Physical Examination	XX	XX			
Preparation and Collection of Specimens	XX	XX	X	X	
Care of Rubber Goods and Use	XX	XX	X	X	X
Fumigation of Rooms	X	X			
Disinfection of Clothing and Bed Linen	X	X			
Disinfection of Excreta	X	X			
Disposition of Sputum in Infectious Diseases	X	X			
Temperature, Pulse and Respiration	XX	XX	X		
Charting	XX	XX			
Sterilization and Care of Instruments	X	X	X		
Foot Bath	XX	XX			
Sitz Bath	XX	XX			
Fomentations	XX	XX	X		
Compresses	XX	XX	X		
Stupes	XX	XX			
Poultices	XX	XX			
Plasters	XX	XX			
Inunction	XX	XX	X		
Inhalation	XX	XX	X		
Preparation for Operation	XX	XX	X		

Binders—Abdominal	XX	XX	X		
Breast	XX	XX			
Preparation of the Patient for the Operating Room	X	X	X		
Care of the Patient upon return from the Operating Room	X	X	X	X	
Enemata—Cleansing	XX	XX	X		
Nutritive	XX	XX			
Oil	XX	XX			
Douches—Vaginal	XX	XX	X		
Aural	X	X			
Nasal	X	X			
Catheterization	X	X			
Enteroclysis	X	X			
Hypodermoclysis	XX	XX			
Lavage	X	X			
Gavage	X	X			
Test Meals	X	X			
Bladder Irrigation	X	X			
Colonic Irrigation	X	X			
Croup Tent	X	X			
Hypodermic Injections	XX	XX			
Gynecological Positions	X		X		
Cupping	XX	X			
Administration of Medicines	XX	X	X		
Gynecological Positions; Preparation for Examination	X	X	X		
Alcohol Sponge	XX	XX			
Temperature Sponge	XX	XX	X		
Pack—Hot, Dry	XX	XX	X		
Hot, Wet	[illegible]	[illegible]	X		
Cold	XX	XX			
Care of the Dead	XX	XX			

REMARKS: Miss Ponsness has shown marked improvement, she works rapidly and does neat, finished work. She is well liked by the patients. Her theoretical work is good.

Elvira L. Grabow R.N. Instructor.

Figures 9A–9B. Record of Nursing Procedures, Louise Ponsness, 1928. From Minnesota Historical Society's Collection #152.K.20.11(B), Box 5, St. Luke's Hospital Records, St. Luke's Hospital Training School for Nurses, Folder: Louise Ponsness.

traditional emphasis on practical learning and experience, a tradition that even today casts doubt on knowledge gained mainly from books. The reality of this situation, and the ongoing struggle to define the nature of nursing, is often brought to awareness in small, easily overlooked ways. For us, one reminder came during a recent visit to a prestigious university school of nursing in the eastern United States. On the way from the airport, Olson shared a taxi with an energetic, self-described "factory nurse" (occupational health nurse) who lived in the same area as the university. The nurse was more than willing to provide her impression of the school of nursing, though she added that she was not a baccalaureate nurse. She explained that, while the university nursing students take an impressive list of courses, the problem is that even after graduation "they can't control the (hospital) unit."[63]

Yet the finely honed skills that transformed a probie into an experienced nurse, with a confidence equal to any skilled artisan, were veiled by the assumption that "skill" was something masculine, both in how it was defined and in who was allowed to attain it.[64] This gave nurses' work a kind of invisibility, and with it a corresponding remarkable freedom to shape their own domain, since what they did was not seen as overlapping or in the way of the masculine jurisdiction of medicine. Invisibility, then, was a mixed blessing for nurses. It was far from unique, being common in other predominately female occupations. For example, a study of clerical workers during the last part of this century revealed "a whole array of positions," from office management to healthcare coordination, in which male supervisors were "full of personal praise" for the women occupying these positions, "but the work itself was never considered."[65] In each instance, it was found, a woman's job responsibilities and accomplishments were hidden under the heading: "low level (female) clerical support."[66]

∿

Although the exact nature of nursing may have been hidden to many outside this field, among the women of St. Luke's it was well understood. For them, nursing meant handling, managing, and controlling individuals, as well as situations, with the aim of producing neat, finished-appearing work. What is glaringly absent from their idea of nursing is the term "caring" and the various words associated with caring that were in common use during this period: "nurturing," "soothing," and "comforting." Instead, "handling," "managing," and "controlling" were the constant terms used to report and assess nurses' work. Ironically in today's perspective, when "care" was mentioned, it was in reference to inanimate things, such as "care of room or ward" or "care of bed and bedding."

Equally unlikely as finding expressions of caring in the conversations and reports of the St. Luke's nurses is trying to find room for their definition of nursing within the current rhetoric of caring. Typical of other accounts in the nursing literature, an article in the *Journal of Nursing Education* claims a historic basis for the following interpretation of caring and, by implication, nursing: "assisting another to grow in a cognitive and emotional sense so that the receiver of the care may become self-actualized."[67] In another recent example, nursing, "the philosophy and science of caring," is depicted as "mental-spiritual growth for self and others; finding meaning in one's own existence and experiences; discovering inner power and control; and potentiating instances of transcendence and self-healing."[68] A frequently cited expert on caring and nursing adds that receptivity is the key to accomplishing these aims, explaining that caring occurs when the nurse "receives the other" (the patient) completely.[69]

In sharp contrast, the definition of nursing that was reinforced year after year among the women of St. Luke's emphasized an approach to nursing that was based in action, force, and pragmatism, not receptivity. To maintain that their view of nursing can be subsumed within contemporary notions of caring, as nursing leaders essentially have tried to do, threatens to enlarge this concept beyond usefulness. Consider, for a moment, the following description of caring and nursing offered by a noted historian of nursing: "an unbounded act, difficult to define, even harder to control."[70] Although an attitude of caring may be implicit in nursing, the St. Luke's nurses would have had difficulty understanding, let alone accepting, such a nebulous expression of nursing action. For them, nursing was neither vague nor uncertain, but a clearly delineated endeavor that embraced physical strength, physical closeness, and physical skill.

No doubt these early nurses would have echoed the sentiment of one contemporary nurse who, frustrated with the present discourse on caring, declares "caring alone is not enough."[71] This same nurse argues that a more suitable view of nursing is one that recognizes that "nurses today . . . must reason well, make deliberative judgments, and speak forcefully."[72] She credits her insight on nursing to the legacy of early-twentieth-century nursing activist Lillian Wald, whom she states took an action-oriented, assertive approach to nursing. As fitting as it may be for present-day nurses, this "new" approach would also seem very familiar to the women of St. Luke's.

Still unexplained, however, is the wide gap between the perception of nursing by early rank-and-file nurses, and the more visible interpretations espoused by nursing leaders and historians. Part of the explanation is that modern claims to caring seem to make intuitive sense, as they build on traditional ideas of femininity. The receptive and nurturing qualities associated with caring emerge from a highly gendered and psychologized interpretation of women's different socialization and social experiences relative to men. Consequently, information to the contrary can be rejected, or at least reframed, if it does not fit preconceived notions. As sociologist Steinberg observes, "The central defining characteristics of jobs are often perceived in terms that are consistent with sex-role stereotypes."[73]

Exploring job perception further, Steinberg takes special note of authority, an aspect of work that is implicit in the St. Luke's terms of handling, managing, and controlling. She asserts, "Authority is part of the male sex role, and everyone sees the authority associated with male work, while the authority associated with female work is invisible."[74] For nurses, most of whom are women, work such as handling, controlling, and managing thus remains hidden, obscured by explanations that seem to have a better fit with accepted beliefs about work and gender.

Arguments that a receptive and nurturing caring is the historic essence of nursing also stem from nursing leaders today identifying this concept as the focal point of their field's special knowledge. "One of the most consistent strategies to achieve professionalization for nursing," explains a nurse sociologist, "has been the attempt to acquire a unique knowledge base, the possession of such knowledge being seen as one of the essential traits of a 'true' profession."[75] And yet, while prominent nurses, particularly those in academia, continue to promote the centrality of caring, they have consistently acted to distance nurses earning baccalaureate and graduate degrees from direct participation in providing such care.

A dean emeritus of one of the nation's foremost schools of nursing acknowledges that "the vast majority of nurses with university education have either no or limited contact in the health services with patients."[76] Nonetheless, this fact does not deter him from asserting, along with numerous other nursing leaders, that entry into nursing practice should be at the doctoral level, rather than the current system in which individuals may enter with a two-year degree, a three-year hospital diploma, or a baccalaureate degree.[77] While this assertion might be effective as a professionalizing strategy, it runs the risk of condoning the idea that nurses are a small and elite group that, by definition, does not deliver nursing care but coordinates it and provides backup through advanced knowledge and skills.[78]

An associate dean at another leading school of nursing confirms that "the functions for nursing as a member of the health care team have moved away from being primarily the provider of total patient care to manager of the delivery of care."[79] The resultant deskilling of nursing means that university-educated nurses are frequently in the position of just arranging for nursing to be done by others, most of whom are minimally qualified nursing assistants, rather than doing the work themselves. The irony of this situation was recently depicted in a *Better Homes and Gardens* cartoon in which a nurse tells a patient, "The doctor's nurse's aides' assistant can see you now."[80]

Not only does the notion of a singular tradition of caring clash with the experience of the St. Luke's nurses, but the dedication to a psychological caring ideal by nursing leaders is doubtful, given their repeated calls for reforms that would only widen the gap between nurses and patients. Caring, as understood in both the past and the present, could simply be one of several unspoken traditions that have been handed down to succeeding generations of nurses, a part of nursing that, as some contend, is "unrecordable and hence not entirely legitimate."[81] To rely on this part to define the whole, though, particularly in regard to understanding nursing history, tends to cloud other meanings of nursing, especially those in evidence among ordinary nurses. In fact, the persistence of disparate meanings and traditions helps to explain the deep divisions that continue to plague nursing in the United States, divisions that preclude agreement on even the basic issue of what preparation one must have to be called a nurse.

For the women of St. Luke's, caring was a subtext to a definition of themselves and their work that challenges traditional ways of viewing women in general, and nurses in particular, in the past. Handling the sick, managing other workers, and controlling the ward, all to produce neat, finished-appearing work, were responsibilities that held consistent to the nurses' frequently stated ideals of physical and mental stamina and skill. In addition, the fact that practical learning was not sacrificed to service at St. Luke's, as historians have previously argued was normative, fit with the apprentices' expectations about mastering nursing techniques through an extended period of hard work and training. At the same time, the emphasis on hands-on experience versus book learning and theory matched the women's belief that common sense and practical ability were more important than intellect and scholastic talent.

To this point, however, we've considered the women as one group, regardless of whether or not they completed the nursing program. In general, all the nurses seem to have shared common expectations and heard similar messages about their chosen field, as well as having faced the same arduous schedule of work and training. Of course, this begs the question of why some left training early while others remained until graduation. Most importantly, what do the experiences of those who left early suggest about the image of nursing that has begun to emerge from St. Luke's? These questions are the focus of the next chapter.

6

Grounds for Dismissal, Reasons to Leave

I wanted to tell you I am not coming back (to training). . . . I'm
beastly sorry after all you have done things turned out this way,
but I guess it couldn't be helped.

—St. Luke's trainee, ca. 1920[1]

A s the 1920s dawned, some of the most significant social changes of
the century were underway, including women's suffrage, prohibition, and social service. Renowned nursing educator Mary Adelaide Nutting reflected, "Prohibition and woman suffrage are two of the
recent great social movements which will profoundly affect the future of
nursing."[2] Inspired by the changes sweeping the nation, St. Paul nurses
joined with other area women in establishing public drinking fountains
throughout the city, organizing Children's Health Days, and providing
fresh milk for children through milk stations they set up in the schools.[3]
Many of the St. Luke's trainees, feeling the buoyant mood of the new
decade, no doubt tackled their work with rekindled zeal. They were likely
encouraged also by the January 1920 agreement to raise private-duty nursing fees by "five dollars per week in all cases, with five hours off duty each
day."[4]

Some trainees, however, must have found it difficult to appreciate the
widespread optimism. By choice, circumstance, or some combination of the
two, these women faced an untimely end to their training. One such individual, Miss Edythe Tanner, wrote to the superintendent of nursing, on July
9, 1920: "Miss Patterson, you will find enclosed under separate cover, the
textbooks, property of St. Luke's Hospital, which I am returning. Also the
uniform and cap which are the only articles of uniform I happened to have,

which did get mixed with my belongings. I can assure you they are of no value whatever to me and I am only too glad to return them."[5] Miss Tanner had been a St. Luke's nurse for just over two years. One can imagine that the indignation apparent in her message was evident also in her face as she delivered the note and closed the door of the hospital behind her for one last time. She had a relatively short walk to the central train station, where she then boarded the coach to her hometown of Little Falls, Minnesota.

The events surrounding Miss Tanner's early departure from the hospital were at once unique, yet similar to those involving the 298 other individuals who left St. Luke's prior to completing their training. Like many of these women, Miss Tanner's interest in nursing was initially sparked by hearing about friends and relatives who were nurses. Her decision to apply to St. Luke's followed conversations with a friend who previously graduated from the hospital.

Miss Tanner had been far from a novice when it came to the actual work of nursing, having accumulated ten months of nursing experience in another hospital prior to entering St. Luke's in April 1918. Although her file gave no clue as to why she left her former position, the work records of all the applicants show that prior training experience was not unusual. In any event, the descriptions of Miss Tanner reveal that her work and training at St. Luke's progressed satisfactorily until the morning of February 23, 1919. On that morning, according to the nursing superintendent, "Miss Tanner, a night nurse, refused to . . . return to the birth room after breakfast to assist putting same in order for the day nurses as is customary in the regular routine of the hospital."[6] This was only the beginning of her difficulties.

Alerted by this incident, the nursing superintendent, Sarah Higgins, began to pay closer attention to Miss Tanner's work. Her concern grew, through her own observations of the apprentice and discussions with other supervisors. Miss Higgins made particular note of the following problems, some of which were clearly more serious than others:

· Miss Tanner neglected a patient's hair. The hair, which was long and heavy, was not combed for a week, and was very much snarled and matted.
· On night duty, I often found her sitting at the desk reading . . .
· While on the Ground Floor . . . she refused to go to the attic for a cot bed, saying that she had just been once, and that it was orderly's work anyway.
· She stayed at a friends over night one Saturday night without permission, and when brought to task about it, she claimed that she did not know it was against the rules.

· She came to take three late (for duty) permissions in one week—only two were allowed. . . . Of course, it is quite possible that she did forget, but it is very unusual for the nurses to forget anything of that sort.[7]

Despite differing levels of urgency and significance, however, the standards of the time dictated that none of these problems could be taken lightly. The first duty of a night nurse, for example, was to ensure that patients were properly attended to, rather than spending time reading. Staying out late, unsupervised, could cast aspersions on nurses who were already perceived to be morally threatened by the relative independence provided by working for pay outside the home. Just as troubling, Miss Tanner's refusal to carry out instructions upset a system that depended on orders being given and carried out, not only from nurse to nurse, but between nurses and other groups such as physicians and ancillary staff. Still, it was another difficulty that created the most tension.

While on night duty in June 1920, the superintendent wrote,

Miss Tanner took a doctor's order for Morphine for a very sick child of three years. The doctor said that he ordered Morphine grs. 1/64th, and she wrote the order Morphine grs. 1/6 to 1/4. Fortunately, there was a special nurse on with the child, and she knew better than to give such a dose to a child. Miss Tanner did not report her mistake in taking down the doctor's order either to the head nurse or to me. . . . Any junior nurse—Miss Tanner is a senior—should know better than to give that amount of Morphine to a child.[8]

Whether seen from the vantage point of the past or present, this was a grievous error that threatened the patient's health and the nurse's credibility. As a result, the entire situation was documented in great detail and extensively discussed among nursing supervisors. It was also brought to the attention of the Training School Committee, a group of three graduate nurses and three hospital officials who oversaw the functioning of the program.[9] Their lengthy review focused on the obvious possibility of death had the large dose of morphine been given. In all of the discussions, the error was also viewed in light of the fact that Miss Tanner was now a senior or third-year nurse. She was seen as an experienced apprentice, for whom higher, more stringent expectations were the rule.[10]

According to usual arguments, any one of Miss Tanner's previous infractions should have resulted in immediate dismissal, and if by some rare chance her initial difficulties were overlooked, she certainly should have been asked to pack her bags after the medication incident. "No tolerance of student misconduct was allowed," explain historians Kalisch and

Kalisch.[11] Even inconsequential offenses such as having "grumbled at the least extra duty . . . or question(ing) the rules," observes an expert on nursing history in the Midwest, would prompt a nurse to be "quickly dismissed as a 'troublemaker.'"[12] Or as stated by another historian, "Most students who left training were dismissed, without hearing, for minor rule infractions."[13] This "repressive discipline," claimed the author of the classic volume *American Nursing,* was "a necessary attribute of 'training.'"[14]

Yet no single problem alone prompted Miss Tanner's early departure. Instead, she was dismissed only after numerous difficulties, along with the failure of repeated attempts at remediation. For instance, after her first infraction, in which she "neglected a patient's hair . . . for a week," she "was made to take her off duty time and clear out the hair, which was a task of several hours."[15] The three infractions that followed resulted in three months suspension, with the understanding that Miss Tanner would use the time to reflect on her choice of occupation. She was being encouraged to leave but not forced to leave.

Shortly after returning to duty following this hiatus, the "late permissions" situation finally brought the possibility of dismissal to the fore. Even then, however, the superintendent pondered, "Are we justified, in view of her past history, in expelling her from the Training School for such a trifling offense, or would it be wiser to pass the matter over with the usual punishment?"[16] In the ensuing discussions with the other nursing supervisors and members of the Training School Committee, a consensus was reached, caution prevailed, and Miss Tanner was given another chance to complete her training.

"The question of expelling her . . . was (again) debated" following the morphine incident. In a move that must have caused some uneasiness in the apprentice, she was brought before the nursing superintendent and a member of the Training School Committee "and carefully questioned."[17] Finally the decision went against Miss Tanner and she was dismissed from the program. Perturbed by a reminder to return all items of uniform prior to leaving the hospital, she left, undaunted, after handing the superintendent the indignant note described above.

The events involving Miss Tanner contradict usual beliefs about how problems with trainees were dealt with. In particular, the detailed descriptions of her difficulties challenge the generally accepted idea that specific reasons for dismissal were seldom given. Nor did her situation fit with the common assertion that "instant dismissal, even in the last days of a student's final year" followed quickly on the heels of even minor violations, "such as leaving the hospital without permission."[18] Rather, Miss Tanner committed recurrent offenses of varying levels of severity over an extended period. Moreover, the final decision to dismiss her came only after a series of consultations, meetings, and soul-searchings, along with attempts to rectify the situation. It was neither an abrupt or arbitrary decision, but one that was arrived at through a careful and deliberate process.

Was Miss Tanner's situation unique? Was she treated differently, perhaps because of an especially benign group of supervisors at the time, or because she was thought to somehow merit special treatment? Others left the hospital before graduation, too, though substantially fewer than previous arguments would lead us to expect.[19] Most importantly, the records of this group of just over one-third (35.7 percent) of all St. Luke's nurses provided ample opportunity to explore the questions surrounding the early departure of Miss Tanner and others.

~

Among the individuals who did not complete training, there was a nearly even split between those who were dismissed and those who resigned. These two subgroups were not equal, however, in terms of how their members were looked upon by others. While nurses like Miss Tanner endured considerable reproach, and had their files marked "left involuntarily," the same was not true for nurses who "left voluntarily," or resigned. Thus, when Lila Greene wrote in 1930, "Please accept my resignation, it shall not be possible for me to return and complete my training at St. Luke's Hospital for several years perhaps," she received a cordial good-bye and the assurance that she was welcome to return.[20] As the use of the term "resignation" further attests, even in leaving, the language of training was closer to work or apprenticeship than school.

The exact reasons for not completing the training program, whether voluntarily or involuntarily, result of dismissal or resignation, add depth to the picture of nursing work and training at St. Luke's. The reasons given fall into distinct categories according to the events involved, and they were also defined in terms of whether they were the primary cause of leaving, or a less important, secondary cause. As in Miss Tanner's situation, there was often more than one factor that brought a premature end to training. An even closer look at her records reveals that her difficulties in working with patients, epitomized by the medication incident, were the main reasons for her dismissal. Her problems "off-duty" were less important, secondary influences.

Specific reasons were listed for more than nine out of ten (93.0 percent) of the women who did not graduate from St. Luke's. This included 278 nurses, a surprisingly high number given that nursing historians have gener-

Table 5. Primary Reason for Not Completing Training (in %)*

	1897–1910	1911–1923	1924–1937	All
Dissatisfied	20.3	22.2	16.8	19.4
Physical	31.1	20.0	18.4	22.3
Personality	5.4	7.8	6.1	6.5
Practical Work	14.9	21.1	18.4	18.3
Theory	2.7	0	11.4	5.4
Family and Marriage	18.9	26.7	21.9	22.7
Natural Ability	4.0	0	2.6	2.2
Breaking the Rules	2.7	2.2	4.4	3.2
Number of Nurses	74	90	114	278

Source: see Table 1.
*Percentages are based on 93.0% (278) of those who did not complete training and for . whom reasons were available.

ally argued that scant attention was paid to documenting dismissals and resignations. When explanations were provided at other institutions, these same observers add, vague references to a "troublesome" or "unfit" nurse took the place of precise descriptions.[21] In contrast, the St. Luke's records include relatively detailed explanations for any abrupt or unexpected ending to training, including, as mentioned, both primary and secondary factors.

The primary reasons that nurses did not graduate comprise eight general problem areas (see table 5), with the majority (82.7 percent) falling into four categories: dissatisfied, physical problems, difficulties with "practical work," and family and marriage issues.[22] A similar pattern was revealed when primary and secondary reasons were combined (see table 6). In comparing all of the reasons with the number of nurses involved, the totals indicate that more than one factor for not completing the program frequently was cited. Moreover, the steady rise in the likelihood of additional reasons being given suggests that problematic situations were scrutinized with increasing diligence over time.

Common Concerns

"Dissatisfied" nurses expressed a range of dislikes, along with distinct preferences. The largest number would have agreed with Hildegard Stanger. She left St. Luke's in 1924 because, as she told the nursing superintendent,

Table 6. Primary and Secondary Reasons for Not Completing Training (in %)*

	1897–1910	1911–1923	1924–1937	All
Dissatisfied	18.6	15.7	13.0	15.0
Physical	28.6	18.4	16.7	19.6
Personality	7.7	12.9	8.4	8.4
Practical Work	15.4	23.8	25.6	23.0
Theory	3.3	2.0	10.7	6.4
Family and Marriage	17.6	19.7	15.8	18.8
Natural Ability	3.3	1.4	3.3	2.6
Breaking the Rules	5.5	6.1	6.5	6.2
Total Reasons	91	147	215	453

Source: see Table 1.

*Percentages are based on 93.0% (278) of those who did not complete training and for whom reasons were available. Number of nurses in each period is the same as Table 5.

"I do not like to be with sick people."[23] Miss Stanger reached this conclusion quickly, because she left after only five days in training. This quick departure from the program was closer to the norm for those who left early than the two-years plus that Miss Tanner spent in training. Close to two-thirds (62.2 percent) of the apprentices who did not graduate left before six months, four out of five (80.6 percent) before the first year ended.

Dissatisfaction occasionally involved other aspects of training as well. Eleanor Bjerke, for example, left after only one day, stating that she "did not like the Nurses' Home."[24] Flora Quimby stayed much longer, nearly one and one-half years, but finally resigned on April 18, 1932, in part, because "the hours on duty are too long."[25] When she later asked to transfer to Immanuel Hospital, her objection to the work schedule was discussed by the superintendents of nursing at St. Luke's and Immanuel. "As far as hours of duty are concerned," explained the St. Luke's superintendent, "we have an eight hour duty day and night . . . we feel that the length of hours should not be a hardship," in what was a common exchange of information between nursing officials from different hospitals and training programs.[26] Despite the concern shared, St. Luke's gave her a favorable recommendation, including the observation that "she is capable of doing nice bedside nursing," and Immanuel accepted her into its program.[27] She had a second chance at another hospital.

"I do not like the work," was often used by an additional group of women who stated clearly the alternatives they hoped to pursue. Three trainees, for example, expressed their disillusionment with nursing and then stated their intention "to take up music."[28] Another trainee entered St. Luke's in 1917, but resigned the following year after noting that she preferred "to go on with college education" rather than to continue nurses' training. Among her supervisors, there was little surprise or dismay, since they had previously remarked that she "did not seem fitted for the work of a nurse."[29] There was considerable regret, however, when a "competent, reliable, and desirable" nurse from Amery, Wisconsin, resigned from the hospital in 1916 because "she decided she preferred to teach."[30]

Their nursing experiences obviously left these women dissatisfied, but not downtrodden or broken. When Lillian Gray decided to end her training after she had devoted herself to the work of nursing for three and a half months, it was because she "thought she wasn't being used right."[31] In early September of 1910, she abruptly resigned, pausing only long enough to leave this brief message for the nursing superintendent: "I think Miss Miller (a senior nurse) quite unjust to report me when . . . I told her I didn't feel competent to do Mr. Thomas' dressing. Everything belonging to the hospital in my possession is in the dresser drawer."[32]

Equally determined, a 1921 probationer did not even stop to write a message after a meeting with the superintendent of nursing left her feeling slighted and indignant. The superintendent explained: "On the morning of June 17th, she came to me and demanded . . . to know if I was going to keep her on. I reproved her for her manner and she was most rude. She went immediately to the home and packed her trunk. I sent over for her but she refused to come to the office and left at once."[33] In this individual's file, like most of those represented in this category, the superintendent marked, "resigned."

The impression of self-possessed decisionmakers that seems to characterize these trainees at St. Luke's was reinforced by women who bravely expressed their disillusionment with training and subsequently left for other endeavors.[34] Of course, skeptics might argue that it was precisely these strong-willed women who would have resigned, leaving less confident and less forceful women behind. Such analysis would support the belief that "institutional norms weighed in favor of submission . . . (and) self-abnegation."[35] A pattern, intentional or not, of winnowing out strong-willed women would certainly cast a shadow on the image of nurses and nursing that has emerged thus far. It is therefore important to ascertain the existence and extent of other reasons for leaving.

Unlike those who resigned to pursue interests outside of nursing, individuals whose "physical problems" became a major impediment to their work in the hospital seldom had any other choice but to leave training. "We both know nursing is a strenuous piece of work even for the most strong," explained Grace Scott, the superintendent of nurses from 1930 to 1934.[36] Miss Scott was trying to soften the blow of dismissal for a nurse who "seemed to find bedside nursing very difficult." The nurse's problem was attributed to a general "lack of physical strength and stamina."[37]

"Left hospital—unable to continue—not strong," is the brief note that described one nurse's early departure in 1907.[38] A similar fate befell another woman who, despite three years prior experience as an "office nurse," left in 1913 "as she found the practical work too hard."[39] Still another was "obliged to leave" in 1921 because she had "very little stamina and . . . perseverance."[40] Although the exact wording of the various explanations changed slightly from individual to individual, the underlying emphasis on strength and endurance remained unchanged from the program's earliest years to its last. For at least one graduate, interviewed in the late 1980s for this study, this definition of nurses as a group selected for strength stayed with her for the half-century since her own graduation. During the interview, she made a point of sharing two lines from Shakespeare that she had carried with her since training:

> The weakest kind of fruit
> Drops earliest to the ground.[41]

For some, weakness was attributed to an obvious impairment, rather than a general lack of strength and stamina. Foot problems were particularly common in this regard. For example, the explanation of why Fannie Hoard left after only a month was both figuratively and literally true: "Unable to stand work. Trouble with feet."[42] A head nurse summarized the plight of another woman with an equally matter-of-fact observation: "she was handicapped by being very small and slight."[43] Similar comments were made about individuals who had "a weak back" or "lack(ed) a strong physique."[44]

A devastating illness was even more likely than any specific impairment to abruptly end an apprentice's work and training. Before antibiotics existed, when immunology was in its infancy, those who toiled at patients' bedsides day after day were more vulnerable than we might realize today.[45] Even before entering training, a large percentage of the women (42.1 percent) reported having had at least one episode of "serious sickness." Scarlet fever topped the list, followed by diphtheria, pneumonia, bronchitis, catarrhal jaundice (infectious hepatitis), smallpox, malaria, typhoid, tuberculosis, spinal meningitis, and infantile paralysis (poliomyelitis).[46]

No wonder that many of the women fell prey to these same diseases during their apprenticeship, at least if usual accounts of nursing's past are accepted. Beyond simple exposure to sickness, nurses who were overworked were more at risk than those with manageable workloads of developing illness. Historian and nursing leader Isabel Stewart explained, "School records do not indicate how many nurses were actually incapacitated, but survivors tell many tales of lives lost and lifelong invalidism incurred by overwork and what seems now a criminal neglect of health. These and other strains and hazards associated with the nurses' training were accepted not only as the inevitable casualties of the war against a disease but as a necessary part of the toughening process."[47] Indeed, there is evidence that physical "toughening" was considered a natural part of training at St. Luke's. In one instance in 1910 a woman was labeled "a very weak sister" after missing over four months due to "a gastric ulcer and chronic gastric disturbance."[48] Presumably, nurses were expected to quickly overcome such problems or endure them while still carrying out their work. Unable to meet either expectation, the apprentice "was not taken back in training."

This seems consistent with expectations at other area nursing programs. Recalling her turn-of-the-century training at a neighboring hospital, Matilda Lindstrom observed, "The summers of 1900 and 1901 two severe epidemics of typhoid struck . . . seven of our nurses got down with typhoid fever. Five of them died. Hannah Johnson and Edith Johnson who entered training in 1899 never graduated. They died in the epidemic. . . . I think a special tribute should have been paid the two nurses. They never said they were feeling ill, took their own temperatures, kept mum until their temperatures reached 105°F, worked all those days."[49] Not only were selflessness and toughening integral parts of nursing—the underlying message of this account—but "work in the sick room" increased the vulnerability of nurses to illness. This last fact was further illustrated, and in an equally dramatic manner, during the 1918–1919 outbreak of Spanish influenza, "America's forgotten pandemic."[50]

In St. Paul and Minneapolis, along with other cities and towns hard struck by the devastating outbreak of influenza, citizens "suffer(ed) severely."[51] Many were observed to simply "drop dead on the sidewalks."[52] Even with a massive mobilization of physicians and nurses, the national death total exceeded 450,000.[53] To compound this problem, "in the fall of 1918, (while) the pestilential flu was sweeping the country, leaving suffering and broken homes in its wake, Minnesota suffered . . . the worst catastrophe in its history—a forest fire."[54] The rapid fire swept over 1,500 square miles in the northern part of the state, leaving 432 people dead and thirteen thousand people homeless.

Nurses from around Minnesota, including those from St. Luke's, struggled to combat the ravages of illness and fire, and in the process "beheld the acme of human misery."[55] "Facing the enemies canon at the battlefront," one nurse explained, "was not as courageous nor hazardous a deed" as tending to the hundreds of Minnesotans who were now sick. No sooner had the fires died up north, then the thousands of survivors were "stricken with grief, (made) helpless with flu, while pneumonia and smallpox were rampant."[56] Tragedy begat trauma.

Throughout the state, hospitals were filled beyond capacity, prompting the city of St. Paul to open a "free influenza hospital of 300 beds to care for urgent cases."[57] Prominent city businesses, including the St. Paul Gas Light Company and American Hoist and Derrick, requested face masks for all of their employees. On Summit Avenue, the city's most fashionable address, well-heeled women created a stir by wearing chiffon veils as masks to a tea. Across the river, in Minneapolis, a panicked press blamed an upsurge in influenza patients on "fake peace news" that had sent thousands of people into the streets to celebrate what they mistakenly believed was the end of World War I.[58]

Without a doubt, the risk of illness among nurses was greatly heightened during this period. One writer, who chronicled the effects of the influenza outbreak at a military camp in Massachusetts, reported that at its peak there were more than fifteen hundred new cases per day, with mortalities of 27 percent among officers, 40 percent among enlisted men, and 33 percent among nurses.[59] Although exact mortality rates were not available for nurses at St. Luke's or other Minnesota hospitals, anecdotal evidence suggests a similarly baneful situation.

In December 1918, Ruth Eaton, a St. Luke's nurse who was recovering at home from "trouble with my heart," wrote to the superintendent of nursing inquiring whether "the epidemic among the nurses has been stopped?"[60] Unfortunately, the answer was no. The deaths of at least two of Miss Eaton's coworkers and friends, in December 1918 and May 1919, were a direct result of the outbreak of influenza.[61]

Frightened by the deaths of nurses as well as patients, another apprentice left the hospital suddenly and without notifying the superintendent when she felt herself becoming ill. The nurse's sister later wrote to St. Luke's, apologizing for her sibling's action. The sister remarked, "We all feel *dreadfully* [original emphasis] to think she left the Hospital as she did . . . she was not well—in fact I think it is only during the last week or ten days that she has commenced to feel more like herself, more as she did before she had the Flu."[62] It was understood that quality nurses somehow did not succumb to illness, at least not to the point of letting it interfere with their patient care.

Nursing certainly involved difficult and hazardous work, as well as a belief in toughening, but at St. Luke's there seems little if any basis for historian Stewart's accusation of "criminal neglect of (nurses') health."[63] In fact, increasing scrutiny and concern about nurses' health led to a steady decrease in the percentage of women who left training due to physical problems (see tables 5 and 6).[64] Of course, closer scrutiny was in the hospital's interest, both in terms of screening out unsuitable applicants and in limiting the effects of illness and disability on those already in training. Greater attention to health also paralleled general advances in medicine.

For more than two decades, entering nurses were given a perfunctory physical examination that tended to be summarized in a single phrase. Women who appeared fit were described as "of sound and robust constitution"; "the appearance of health and vigor"; "strong and robust and of pleasing appearance"; or "not of the dainty kind."[65] Descriptions of those considered to have "defects" were even briefer, such as "short stature"; "a large mouth"; and "bunions."[66]

As a more disciplined and analytic approach began to take hold within the field of medicine, systematic physical examinations for nurses became the norm at St. Luke's. By 1918, this included thorough screenings both prior to and during training.[67] As a result, more women were disqualified during the application process. Others, however, benefited from having potentially career-ending problems identified and remedied. This is perhaps best illustrated by the increasing attention paid to an aspect of anatomy considered crucial to success in nursing—that is, healthy feet. In a typically detailed summary involving a probationer, the examining physician noted: "Feet stand up very well, has a good arch, practically no pronation and the tendo Achilles are a little above right angle. She complains of a little prickling of the ball of the foot in the morning but this appears to be in good position and practically no depression of the anterior arch. Has a mild formation of callouses over the small toe. Advised to get a pair of Mr. Fabel's shoes and wear them as they are."[68]

The steady decline in physical problems among the nurses, along with a greater concern about preventive health measures, not only belies charges of neglect, but also undermines historical claims of abuse. Such claims range from the belief that "exhaustion" was the leading reason for student withdrawals, to the assertion that training conditions worsened over time.[69] Still, challenging these misconceptions does not alter the realization that nursing at St. Luke's, as elsewhere, was always physically demanding and occasionally even perilous. Women who lacked either strength or stamina were unlikely to succeed as nurses.

~

Concerns related to a nurse's "practical work" followed close behind issues of dissatisfaction and illness or disability in bringing about an untimely end to training. Like the definition of nursing at St. Luke's, these concerns involved the full array of problems that could arise in how a woman "handled patients" or "managed the floor." One young woman, whose practical work had been criticized by senior apprentices and regular staff, left the hospital in 1910, just ahead of an anticipated dismissal. With a directness characteristic of the era, the superintendent of nurses offered the following explanation:

> She was careless, incompetent and was not trustworthy. I finally found that she had not given a treatment properly, and told her then that I thought of suspending, or dismissing her, but had decided to give her one more chance, but that she would be dismissed for the first offence. She left that night without waiting to take that chance. She was a year under age but seemed so well developed that I thought she would get along nicely, but was disappointed.[70]

When the same woman later sought to enter the University of Minnesota Hospital, the nationally known superintendent of that program, Louise Powell, contacted St. Luke's. After an exchange of cordialities and a brief discussion of the applicant's potential, the St. Luke's superintendent repeated her previous assessment of the nurse. Aware of the overriding importance of practical work, Miss Powell later wrote that "we have not accepted the (nurse's) application."[71]

As previously mentioned, heads of separate nursing programs often shared information regarding apprentices and graduate nurses. Within the hospital, too, concerns about a particular nurse generally led to discussions among various individuals. This included hospital and nursing superintendents, graduate supervisors, senior apprentices, and, depending on the severity of the situation, the Training School Committee. As in the case of Miss Tanner (described at the start of the chapter) problems with practical work usually ended up before the committee, a clear indication that such problems warranted the highest concern.

After gathering information from several supervisors, Elizabeth Myers, the nursing superintendent in 1924, felt compelled to bring the situation of a "junior nurse" to the attention of the Training School Committee. In a detailed report, Miss Myers explained that "at the time of acceptance (the nurse's) work on the floors . . . was as satisfactory as that of the average nurse at this time, but she was also advised . . . about her incessant talking."[72] More serious problems soon began to occur. Among these, Miss Myers emphasized the following:

· In July, during (the nurse's) term of night duty, I spoke to her about a mistake she had made in medication. She replied that she did not know very much about the drugs she was giving. . . .
· (The nurse) also told one of Dr. Greene's patients, that in her opinion, Dr. Greene only doped his patients and kept them in the hospital too long. . . . The head nurse informed me, stating that she thought I should know. I myself questioned the patient, and she told me that (the nurse) had discussed various patients with her, and their ailments. She said that she did not care to have (the nurse) in her room, and rather than ring for something she really required, went without it, in order to keep her out of the room.
· Patients have also complained of (the nurse's) inconsiderate handling of them. One patient, a woman 83 years of age, asked me to keep her off the floor as long as she was a patient on that floor.[73]

From the standpoint of the women and men who were charged with overseeing the program, the ongoing and serious nature of the problems left no alternative but to "send the nurse packing." In a unanimous decision, she was officially dismissed by the Training School Committee.[74]

More than a story of unfortunate circumstances, the situation of this nurse, and the many others similar to it, challenge several widely accepted beliefs about nursing's past. For instance, the exceeding care with which difficulties were documented at St. Luke's contradicts charges that specific reasons for dismissal were usually not given. Familiar accounts argue otherwise, for instance, that "disloyal or . . . untruthful" was as detailed an explanation as a trainee could expect.[75] Those accounts also argue "minor rule infractions" were more likely to bring a sudden end to training than were "incidents compromising patient safety," yet the particular attention given to concerns involving practical work discredits that notion."[76] Similarly, the ongoing and repeated nature of difficulties that led eventually to dismissal from St. Luke's refutes the often-heard suggestion that school officials tended to punish and dismiss in a capricious and arbitrary manner.

At a minimum, it is clear that a woman's failure to complete training at

St. Luke's, whether forced or not, was seen as a highly important matter that deserved careful attention. This applied to the full range of practical work issues, as exemplified here by a representative collection of comments, each from a different supervisor:

- she was exceedingly clumsy and awkward about her work with the patients.
- throughout training (she) was unruly (and) untrustworthy . . . finally dismissed for going away and remaining out all night after she had been told to be in readiness for an emergency operation.
- she was very untidy, both in work and appearance.
- dismissed on account off [*sic*] being unkind and neglected a patient who was very ill an [*sic*] died the day following.
- while (scheduled for) night duty left . . . without permission, which is against the rules and returned much intoxicated at 7 P.M., and was unable to go on duty. . . . This was not her first offense.
- *Too Slow!*
- she was apparently a good, conscientious girl, but was absolutely unfitted for the vocation of nurse. We were not able to teach her to do the simplest procedures properly . . . (she) failed utterly in anything calling for any real thinking.[77]

These comments, which spanned nearly the entire time the program existed, also covered a range of issues, from the physical skill of handling patients and doing procedures, to matters of speed, neatness, and trust. Serious problems in any of these areas threatened the ultimate goal of doing "finished appearing work," so special attention was devoted to documenting them and intervening, even with dismissal, if warranted. This was not so unusual, however, since the focus on skilled practical work among individuals who did not complete training was consistent within the program as a whole.

～

To explain her abrupt departure from the hospital in 1913, Ruth Richardson wrote, "I've decided to go West with my parents." Besides, she added, "I expect to be married in two years anyway."[78] Although none of the nursing school supervisors wrote in response to Miss Richardson's announcement, there was probably little surprise. After all, concerns involving marriage and family comprised a major category among the reasons why nurses failed to complete training.

While family obligations were the primary motivator for Miss Richardson's resignation, with expectations of marriage only strengthening her resolve, over a third (34.9 percent) of the explanations in this category involved marriage alone. In 1909, for example, Ione Stock "left to be married to an interne (who was) leaving at the same time."[79] Although intimate relationships between physicians and nurses were discouraged, in order to preserve their separate spheres of authority and to avoid losing valued workers, this unwritten rule was ignored on numerous occasions. Of course, the greater stricture was against combining marriage and nursing in general.

For one apprentice, the pressure of concealing her marriage to a childhood sweetheart, and the separation imposed by having to live in the nurses' residence, was simply too much for her to bear. Her resignation, in January 1935, and the disclosure that she had actually married the previous September, likely brought her a sense of relief. Several other apprentices were already aware of the marriage, suggesting the possibility that St. Luke's officials knew, too, but conveniently overlooked an "unfortunate action" by an otherwise productive nurse.[80] In any event, so-called secret marriages occurred with a certain regularity, at St. Luke's and other hospitals, as they did in other fields such as manufacturing.[81]

An illustration from nearby Swedish Hospital also reveals that some women balanced marriage and training, though still in secret. A 1918 graduate of the hospital recalled a situation in which a member of her class "was secretly married and continued nurses' training . . . (while) several of her classmates shared her secret."[82] "Undoubtedly," hospital historians concluded, "there must have been several instances of students marrying 'undercover.'"[83]

Official pronouncements and the strain of maintaining a secret marriage were only partial impediments to a nurse's marrying. As previously noted, marriage bars were common in female-dominated occupations during this era. Such restrictions reflected societal values, by which the pursuit of an occupation outside the home was thought to be incompatible with marriage and raising a family.[84] In addition, during the Great Depression of the 1930s, popular opinion (and federal employment policy) turned against the possibility of there being two wage-earners in a household while others had none. More than one woman seemed to welcome this norm by openly seeking out nursing as a refuge from an unwelcome marriage.[85] Despite occasional efforts to circumvent the prohibition of marriage, not one individual openly questioned this rule at St. Luke's. Such apparent agreement sharply contrasted with the nurses' sometimes outspoken disapproval of other rules, a subject discussed later in this chapter.

Expressing the prevailing view of women in general, and nurses in particular, renowned turn-of-the-century physician William Osler explained, "Marriage is the natural end of the trained nurse; so truly . . . is a woman unmarried, in a certain sense, a woman undone."[86] Numerous social historians have expressed this same idea, though usually in less poetic terms. "The definition of woman" during the early 1900s, concluded one such observer, "maintained the centrality of home and family in women's lives."[87] In fact, societal beliefs in a feminine ideal of marriage and motherhood have extended well beyond the first part of the century, with researchers affirming in a 1960s study that "the prospect of marriage and children permeates every aspect of nursing."[88]

As suggested by these views, reasons for leaving training that focused on broader family concerns were as encumbered by gendered expectations as those that involved marriage alone. Thus, when Marvel Webster openly worried about her mother's worsening illness, in 1923, the superintendent immediately replied that her "first responsibility" was not to continue training, but to be with her mother.[89] Miss Webster registered no surprise at this advice, although it ran against a clearly stated policy prohibiting apprentices from leaving the hospital to "nurse sick relatives at home." In truth, no attempt was ever made to enforce this policy.[90]

For the St. Luke's nurses, both apprentices and supervisors, family concerns were joined by a common thread, sometimes made explicit, other times simply understood, that sexual difference is a "natural" phenomenon that designates women as "the primary tenders of the family."[91] Accordingly, as Miss Webster was leaving to watch over her mother, the superintendent added that she would be permitted to resume training only "if arrangements could be made for some woman to take your place in your mother's home."[92] Not once was the suggestion made that Miss Webster's adult brother or father, who were already living in the family home, might assume responsibility for their family member. Nor did experience in training, which for Miss Webster was less than a year, seem to be a major consideration. Rather, this situation, like many others, reinforced the idea that the illness of a family member became the responsibility of daughters, particularly unmarried ones, rather than sons.

"I entered St. Luke's Training School for Nurses in January, 1913," wrote Clara Clark to the hospital treasurer. She had decided to plead her case directly to the treasurer because of the urgency of her family situation. Miss Clark explained:

> On account of the illness of my Father I was called home in May of that year. The Doctors pronounced his sickness hardening of the arteries. Since that time he has grown more helpless, until now we even have to feed him, also lift him from his chair, it taking both my Mother and myself to do it. . . . I wish to know if there is any possible chance of my obtaining the fifty dollars . . . this money is returned to the nurse at the end of the term, as you probably know. Our financial condition is poor and I had to borrow the money to enter.[93]

She had left before the end of her first term, however, and technically was not entitled to the return of the recently instituted deposit. Yet the treasurer sympathized with Miss Clark's situation. Realizing that she was the only one of her three siblings who was not married, and thus bore the greatest responsibility for helping her parents, he promptly returned the $50.00 and expressed his hope "that you will be able to return to our Hospital."[94]

As Miss Clark's situation further attests, women not only had primary responsibility in tending to sick relatives, but they often took the lead in responding to purely economic tragedies as well. "I have been hesitating to write this letter in hopes that something might turn up to enable me to return to duty this fall," wrote a 1930s nurse from her family's drought-stricken farm in Bruce, South Dakota. However, she explained, "We have had a complete failure in our crops this year; everything has been burned up in the terrible heat and drought making it impossible of returning (sic)."[95] Since her brother was facing a crop failure of his own, the nurse realized that she had no choice but to remain with her parents.

The plight of these nurses underscores the conclusion of feminist historian Evans that even though women of this era were moving away from the strictures of Victorian morality, their individuality was still defined and limited by their gender.[96] Unlike men, women were expected to automatically relinquish or at least forestall occupational plans when marriage loomed or family members experienced hardship. There was a great consistency over time in the marital and family concerns that led to interruptions in training at St. Luke's, demonstrating that, at least in this area, gender-based expectations continued uninterrupted during the program's existence.[97]

ADDED DIFFICULTIES

The remaining factors involved in dismissal and resignation, though less commonly reported, are important to filling in the picture of nursing at St. Luke's. For instance, concerns about an apprentice's personality shed light on both the desirable and undesirable characteristics of a nurse. The portrayal of one individual who resigned in 1922 was typical. She left reluctantly, after a meeting between the nursing superintendent and her older sister, who was also a nurse. According to the notes of the meeting, the superintendent and sister "decided that (the trainee) was wasting her time here, and would better try [*sic*] some other work." As both agreed, the problem was that the trainee "was quiet . . . very reserved (and) did not mix well with other people."[98]

The need for nurses to be forceful and outgoing made personality a target of scrutiny by graduate supervisors and senior nurses. Like the woman just described, concern mounted with an individual who "had no self confidence," or was "very quiet and nervous."[99] "A shrinking little woman" is how one apprentice was labeled just prior to her dismissal.[100] With only slight variation, others left or were asked to leave because they were "too timid to be a strong scrub nurse," "not strong personally," "extremely nervous and self-conscious," or just "unable to carry on—timid and immature."[101] From the perspective of more experienced nurses, such attributes caused individuals to "work with a marked degree of uncertainty," making them unsuitable for nursing.[102]

While a strong personality was valued, however, there was a line beyond which a nurse's temperament might be considered "very aggressive" and consequently problematic.[103] Still, the negativity associated with being an aggressive nurse was minimal when compared to the outright rejection of those who were hesitant or timid. Indeed, evidence of aggressiveness at St. Luke's could only be found in descriptions of women who completed training, not among those of women who left early.

Ardys Kruschke was criticized by a head nurse, in 1925, because she was "inclined to be dictatorial."[104] Yet only months later, at the end of her training, Miss Kruschke was extolled as "a remarkably good nurse, a most dependable and thorough worker . . . kept equipment in good condition . . . a good executive."[105] Certainly effective management of the myriad demands facing a nurse favored strong-willed women. No wonder, then, that such women were likely to succeed in nursing while extremely docile and submissive women were sent packing.

A smaller group of individuals was said to have an "undesirable personality" due, not to a lack of fortitude, but to characteristics that were associated with a "social standing (that) was below average."[106] This last phrase was in reference to a 1907 nurse. In a later example, the hospital superintendent explained to the father of an apprentice that his daughter was "temperamentally unfit" for nursing. The superintendent then explained in more detail when she wrote in the nurse's file: "Her work showed no improvement, and she seemed to be hardly the type of girl that we like for our nurses. The nurses in the home felt that she was rather

common, was loud and rough in her speech, etc. Under these circumstances, we only kept her two of the three months we had placed her on
probation."[107]

In considering social standing, however, a distinct separation was made
between trained nurses and less skilled ancillary personnel, "the help," as
aides and attendants were called. Thus, when one nurse was told that she
had an "undesirable personality and . . . (would) not be taken back in the
Training School," the superintendent offered an alternative. She pointed
out, you "might do very well as an attendant."[108]

Those searching for nursing's academic side among the training program's
concerns are likely to be disappointed. "Theory"—as academic study was
known—was a factor in a relatively small percentage of dismissals and resignations. Foremost on an apprentice's mind, then, had to be her physical,
rather than academic, ability, and her temperament. Even the seeming
increase in attention to theory after 1924 yields to a less obvious, yet more
plausible interpretation.

To begin with, well over half (57.0 percent) of the theory-related difficulties occurred during a brief, four-year span between 1931 and 1935.
Prior to 1931, few problems were reported in this area because, as described
in the preceding chapter, nobody at St. Luke's paid much attention to theory or nurses' academic grades. After 1930, however, a new requirement that
all women had to complete a semester at the University of Minnesota introduced regular grade reports and a uniform number of classroom hours.
Those who failed to earn passing grades in the university courses were
unable to commence hospital training. Suddenly theory was an issue.

What seemed on first glance to represent a major change in St. Luke's
thinking about nursing, however, was merely a pragmatic step during a
time of uncertainty at the hospital.[109] The deepening economic crisis that
gripped the country following the Crash of 1929, with consequent questions about the feasibility of running a training program that met new
demands for academics, meant that the training school committee and
nursing supervisors welcomed the suggestion that coursework be taken
over by the university (with the fee to be paid by trainees). This eased the
burden on St. Luke's to provide classroom instruction for nurses—something they had not equipped themselves to do well—while allowing the
program to function relatively undisturbed.

The relative unimportance of theory versus physical ability or practical
experience emerges clearly in a statistical analysis of an apprentice's prob-

ability of completing training, based on such factors as age, previous education, and occupational, geographic, and religious background. What is revealed, through a process described elsewhere in considerable detail, is that a nurse's previous education had a significantly greater influence than other factors on the likelihood of her graduating from St. Luke's.[110] Although the exact nature of this relationship is consistent with what has been learned so far, it may still cause surprise.

Women who had high school diplomas were far less likely to complete their apprenticeship than women who did not have them.[111] Nurses' success was inversely related to their academic preparation. This is consistent with the scant interest in academic skills at admission and the frequent lapses in tracking academic progress during training. This startling fact seems to confirm nursing historian Melosh's claim of widespread mistrust of theory among rank-and-file nurses.[112] Not only did book learning fail to prepare one for the real work of nursing, it gave rise to difficulties that could spell an end to a nurse's career. Had St. Luke's chosen trainees with more academic preparation, they might have had more difficulty getting nurses to successfully complete their training.

The various findings also help to explain the disappointment and puzzlement expressed by nurses and others with the decision to allow the university to take over classroom instruction. A father expressed his surprise, for example, when he learned that his daughter would not be able to begin hospital training because she had failed several of the university courses. "But we have your signed acceptance for (the) St. Luke's training class," he insisted.[113] Another woman abandoned the idea of training after just a month of classroom instruction. "I discontinue(ed) my courses at the University," she remarked, "because I lost all desire to be a nurse."[114]

~

For a small group of women, it was not their academic ability that was questioned, but their "natural ability. She was "just not fitted for the work" is how the hospital superintendent justified the dismissal of one first-year nurse.[115] "Not suitable to the work" and "not adapted for nursing" were similar criticisms heard of others who were asked to leave the hospital.[116]

Some of the apprentices might have openly wondered about the exact qualities or behavior that prompted such criticism. Was it that they lacked some "womanly characteristic," as various historians have argued?[117] The view of nursing ability as "something inherent in all women" has commonly been part of nursing's "distinctive ideology."[118] As one observer explains, nursing "called forth and used so-called natural aspects of womanhood," such as nurturing and caring.[119] Because these traits are so difficult to define and quantify, they constitute a nebulous margin of error within which a nurse who adequately met all the other criteria could still fail.

While it is possible that womanly qualities were the basis for concerns here, the uncharacteristic lack of detailed rationale, in contrast to other areas of concern, leaves this position inconclusive. The absence of detail actually suggests a lack of importance attached to issues of natural ability and presumed feminine attributes, or perhaps an understanding of those things so hegemonic it did not need to be articulated. The fact that such issues were cited less often than all other issues, however, advances the theory that "natural aspects of womanhood" were considered to be of little consequence to success in nursing.

∼

"Breaking the rules," a phrase used at St. Luke's to refer to the last category of problems, figured prominently in the minds of those outside the hospital, as those within it. Whether it was a positive or negative practice was not so clear. From the first settlements in St. Paul and its environs, one writer remarked, area residents "praised the majesty of the law but often ignored it."[120] As a consequence, temperance societies, the Anti-Cigarette League, and similar organizations were kept busy waging "war on wickedness in Minnesota" throughout the late nineteenth and early twentieth centuries.[121] Citizens heard repeated cautions, such as one to "live simply, without narcotics, animal food or stimulants."[122] And yet the struggles of Minnesotans to embrace moral purity and to conform to the laws of the state were frequently uphill battles. Particularly during the 1920s and 1930s, it seemed the good guys had lost. Prostitution and gambling flourished in the area around St. Luke's, known as Seven Corners, and violence was common throughout the city. In one sensational example, two men and a woman were gunned down in the shadow of the state capitol in what newspapers called "the third outbreak of gang warfare in the Twin Cities within two weeks."[123] Within an easy walk from the hospital, the Green Lantern and numerous other speakeasies did a thriving business, especially during the noon hour.

Rather than combating this situation, St. Paul's police chief, John J. O'Conner, devised a system whereby criminals from across the country were guaranteed safe haven in his city as long as they committed their major offenses elsewhere.[124] The result was the arrival of a succession of public enemies, including Baby Face Nelson, John Dillinger, Alvin Karpis, and Ma and Fred Barker, who routinely sought refuge in St. Paul. Of course, the city could not have remained "gangster ridden" and "a crook's haven" without at least the tacit support of politicians and average citizens.[125] As late as 1933, the leading newspaper in Milwaukee, Wisconsin, pleaded, "It is about time that St. Paul, Minneapolis, and all of Minnesota for that matter, woke up. A complete housecleaning is long overdue. Gangs cannot thrive in a community year after year and ply their trade successfully unless that community is guilty of corruption or the grossest neglect. . . ."[126]

St. Paul nurses joined the fight against lawlessness and depravity, hosting meetings and community activities aimed at reform. Among their efforts was a 1910 discussion that focused on "moral prophylaxis" and culminated in an "urgent request for copies of the pamphlet 'Social Hygiene and the Sexual Plague.'"[127] Those present at the discussion vowed to distribute the material wherever needed. Nurses were also part of a community playground movement that sought "to restore the wholesome influence of family life."[128] By 1912, this woman-led enterprise had helped to create eighty playgrounds and parks in St. Paul.

In this context, "breaking hospital rules" was one of the least common reasons for the dismissal or resignation of a St. Luke's apprentice. After all, it might have been too much to expect strict application of rules since serious transgressions in the larger community were overlooked on a regular basis. Still, the argument that nursing's system of apprenticeship training imposed "severe restrictions" and "prison-like rules" has been a cornerstone of nursing history.[129] Under this system, historians have concluded, nearly every aspect of an individual's life became a potential for disciplinary action, presenting still another obstacle against which nurses had to struggle on the path of professionalization.

Once again, St. Luke's provides a challenge to the normal argument, which is muddied by evidence that only a small number of nurses were charged with rule breaking. At St. Luke's, few nurses failed to complete training due to breaking the rules, but those who did nearly all left as the result of an actual or potential sexual indiscretion, as perceived by nursing supervisors. For instance, the nurse cited at the start of the chapter as being "beastly sorry" for leaving St. Luke's in 1920 tendered her resignation following a sexual relationship while in training and a subsequent infection with "lues" (syphilis). Even so, she was not forced out immediately, however. "I had an offer of work in Minneapolis," the nurse explained, "which would enable me to go to school and take my treatments at the same time."[130]

Years before penicillin became the treatment of choice, the only option for this individual was to endure interventions that were, at best, "moderately effective." It included a series of "Neoarsphenamine-8 intravenous injections interspersed with either Bismuth or Mercury intramuscular injections."[131] Yet as serious as her situation was, and the fact that an important and well-understood rule had been violated, nursing supervisors did not immediately act to dismiss this woman. Instead, she was given several months to formulate her plans, during which time she was described as one who "can use her head to a very good advantage."[132]

The plight faced by this nurse, and similar problems stemming from "ill-conceived relationships," were foremost on the minds of nursing supervisors when formulating and enforcing the rules of training.[133] Sexually transmitted diseases and unintended pregnancies could ruin a young woman's life and lose a good nurse for society. Thus, above all else, they demanded that apprentices live in a nurse's residence and avoid going out past certain hours. Overlooked, whether intentionally or not, was the fact that some women sought sexual fulfillment among their own ranks. "Oh, they roomed together and we knew they were lesbians," explained a St. Luke's graduate during a 1980's interview, in which she discussed relationships among nurses earlier in the century. "But everyone kept it quiet," she added.[134] Perhaps it seemed possible to keep quiet about the illicit homosexual relationships precisely because they were same-sex, and therefore did not cause the same immediate, dire consequences as resulted from illicit heterosexual relationships at the time.

An additional example highlights the veiled discussions that often surrounded incidents of rule breaking and which, after a moment of reflection, reveal implicit concerns about heterosexual impropriety. More than other problem areas, such discussions tended to involve family members as much as the nurse herself. There was nothing unusual, then, when the nursing superintendent in the following situation initially directed her comments about a second-year nurse, named Margaret, to the nurse's mother and older sister. The superintendent pointed out that "Margaret's name has been linked with a group . . . who have admitted frequenting and smoking in a drug store, which we feel is not a desirable place; (she) has also been acting indiscreetly when off duty, and is careless in work."[135]

No further explanation was needed, as the mother responded that her daughter's one-month suspension from training was a reasonable punishment. "She is a very subdued Margaret," the mother added, "and (she) is very sorry for the mistakes she has made and the trouble she has caused you. She has no word of criticism or complaint to offer and hopes that the (training school) committee can see their way clear to take her back at the end of the month."[136] Margaret's sibling followed up with several messages of her own.

"Being Margaret('s) . . . sister," she wrote, "I am very much concerned."

She assured the superintendent that "Margaret has received no sympathy from her home folks for we realize she was treated justly . . . she has not used her 'hours off' to her own best advantage."[137] For her own part, the nurse at first refused to acknowledge that she had broken the rules, providing the following outline of her off-duty activities for "the last six months": "Usually once in two weeks I went to my Aunt's home. Attended Peoples church every Sunday possible; went to an occasional movie; two music concerts, one play; dinners with friends of the family; lunch at Green Gate, Murries, or Schuneman's tea room; one curling game; two basketball games; at Miss Deba's home several times; an occasional date with a boyfriend."[138]

Somewhat later, Margaret admitted to having been in "Donehues Drug Store . . . three or four times." The superintendent replied to the nurse's sister: "According to Margaret's statement, it would seem she has been living the life of any normal girl, but we do know the serious mistakes she has made." Nevertheless, the training school committee accepted the nurse's statement that she had "not wilfully [*sic*] disobeyed any of the rules of the school," noting "we do feel she is worth another trial."[139]

Her return to training was cut short, however, when she was hospitalized at St. Luke's for undisclosed complications following an abortion, performed in a private residence by "a Minneapolis woman."[140] With her indiscretion confirmed, Margaret was required to submit her resignation, in accord with the rules of the hospital and "accepted standards of decency." Despite such serious errors, however, the superintendent later wrote in support of her application to finish training in a Montana hospital. Margaret was described as "a better than average nurse . . . (who) has undoubtedly had ample time to meditate . . . (and) prove to you that she is worthy of the title 'graduate nurse.'"[141]

～

Rather than being subject to tyranny—the common image of training schools—the women who broke the rules at St. Luke's were treated in a cautious and humane manner, similar to the treatment of those who experienced other types of difficulties. There was no evidence of "prison-like rules" or restrictions beyond those gender-based norms generally accepted during this era. Nor was there any indication that the laissez-faire attitude toward law and order, which seemed to pervade parts of the larger community, influenced nursing supervisors or apprentices.

When serious hindrances to training occurred, nurses resigned or were dismissed. In general, the latter action took place only after a pattern of difficulty had developed and corrective measures had failed. From the training program's earliest years to its last, the greatest attention was always reserved for matters that were seen as the core of nursing, that is, the ability to fulfill the pragmatic and highly physical yet skilled demands of this field. While "secret marriages" might be overlooked, poor classroom performance forgotten, and occasional improper behavior tolerated, St. Luke's had no room for women who lacked strength of body or will.

At training's end, those who had succeeded in handling the sick, and in producing neat, finished-appearing work, now descended the steps of the hospital as "graduate nurses." Contemplating their future, no doubt the women were filled with a mixture of both excitement and uncertainty. Exactly what awaited them outside the doors of St. Luke's? The nature of nursing after graduation is the subject of the next chapter.

7

Lasting Impressions

Once a nurse, always a nurse.
St. Luke's nurse, 1989[1]

“I really wanted to be a detective,” Helen Bertsche remarked in 1989, when asked about her decision to become a nurse.[2] Although she was now well into her eighties, the discussion of her old passion for sleuthing made her eyes brighten and her voice rise with an excitement similar to what she must have felt as a young woman. It was the late 1920s again and she was living in her home on the bluffs of St. Paul's West Side, just above the “flats,” a rowdy neighborhood that filled a wide expanse of land that stretched along the Mississippi.

“I always knew when a house in the flats was going up,” Miss Bertsche commented in regard to the increasingly common practice of the late 1920s and 1930s of torching homes and businesses to collect insurance money.[3] Piecing together various clues, she was able to figure out exactly where an arsonist would strike “a day or two before the fire.” Reflecting on this time, she said she now realizes how hard-pressed many people were financially, as the nation's slide into the Great Depression was reflected by a boom in illegal activity in St. Paul. She also recalled one of the most notorious gangsters of this era, Alvin Karpis, who wrote, “Every criminal of any importance . . . made his home at one time or another in St. Paul. If you were looking for a guy you hadn't seen in a few months, you usually thought of two places—prison or St. Paul. If he wasn't locked up in one, he was probably hanging out in the other.”[4] Somewhat wistfully, however, Miss Bertsche pointed out that being a detective was not a realistic ambition for a woman in the late 1920s. With that option closed, she set her sights on nursing, where she relished a different type of challenge. Once she began her work and training at St. Luke's, she never considered turning back. "I wouldn't have left," she insisted, "even to be a detective." As if no other explanation was necessary, Miss Bertsche observed firmly, "Once a nurse always a nurse."[5]

During talks with other St. Luke's nurses, a similar devotion to nursing was repeatedly expressed, although most interrupted their gainful employment for marriage and child rearing. The women of St. Luke's seemed to demonstrate the same degree of zeal and commitment to their work as is often seen among professionals such as physicians, lawyers, and members of the clergy. To explore this finding, and thus to add a final piece to the puzzle of early nursing, this chapter looks closely at the impressions of nursing that the women took with them once their apprenticeship was complete.[6] What did nursing mean to them?

A Congregation of Women

On June 12, 1895, eight young women, all of whom were recent graduates of the St. Luke's Hospital Training School for Nurses, "met for the purpose of organizing an alumani [*sic*] association."[7] Across the continent, alumnae of other training schools were also organizing, prompted by the general uncertainties of work outside the home and the specific demands of private-duty nursing. By 1896, these groups were unified into a single North American association, which became the leading voice for rank-and-file nurses in the United States and Canada: the Nurses' Associated Alumnae.[8]

When members of this major body met at their sixth annual convention, in 1903, one of the last of the famous untrained nurses of the Civil War, Mary A. Livermore, proclaimed with great emotion, "I find all that is within me rising up in this presence . . . a congregation of trained women nurses. Something that in my earlier days I never expected to see."[9] Nursing had come so far in this one woman's lifetime that there was much reason for nurses to feel pride in their chosen occupation. Emotion aside, though, what bound the women together was a pragmatic desire to take hold of their futures. St. Luke's alumnae members had reason to think they were riding the wave of the future when they declared in 1895 that their aim was "to advance in all ways the interests of trained nurses, by meetings, exercises and such corporate action as may tend to that result."[10]

The use of the word "corporate" is telling, as the nation was going through what might be called an incorporation fever at that time. The 1893 World's Columbian Exposition in Chicago is credited with establishing the emergence of corporations and their wealthy leaders as cultural gatekeepers; the fair's commission created the first national corporate alliance of business, culture, and the state.[11] With very different aims from those of corporate business entities like this, the nurses understood that combining efforts was hardheaded practicalism of the sort that would be demanded by the twentieth century. Gone were romanticized notions of nursing, one historian explains, replaced by "the reality of the woman with the scrub brush."[12]

The women of St. Luke's were taught that nursing required an abundance of personal strength, both of mind and body, but they quickly realized that success in their chosen field would demand more than individual strength alone, but also combined strength. Thus, all but one of those who gathered together in 1895 became founding members of the St. Luke's Alumnae Association. They represented half of the fourteen nurses who had completed their training at the hospital in 1894 and 1895.

Yet the women were concerned about more than their own immediate issues. Their aim, "to advance in all ways the interests of trained nurses," expressed an allegiance to a larger nursing community. It was an example of what Reverby has termed "occupational loyalty," a basic consciousness, which she argues "proved difficult to elicit within nursing."[13] The lack of such a consciousness, she further contends, frustrated nurses' "professionalizing and standardizing efforts."[14]

At St. Luke's, however, the nurses had affirmed their connection to nurses in general with their earliest collective statement. Like other historians of nursing, Reverby seems to have missed such expressions of occupational loyalty while focusing on the professionalizing struggles in nursing. The struggles were, indeed, a major interest of nursing's elite, but not of average nurses such as those at St. Luke's. The charge that alumnae associations were narrowly focused on "provid(ing) some kind of mutual benefit society for graduates," in contrast to "organiz(ing) nurses for collective action," suggests that these goals were mutually exclusive.[15] In fact, however, they were not.

A close look at the issues that concerned the St. Luke's nurses confirms that the type of occupational loyalty present among the women was consistent with their training. They focused on matters of practical rather than academic concern, ranging from a hiring protest to Red Cross volunteering. Immediate or "home hospital" issues were uppermost in their minds, yet a review of more than sixty alumnae meetings shows that broader occupational issues were of enduring interest as well (see table 7).[16]

~

Home hospital issues encompassed a range of topics that were both immediate and tangible. For instance, organizational activities focused on tasks commonplace to formal associations, such as approval of members, discussion of

Table 7. Alumnae Interests

Home Hospital Issues		Broader Occupational Issues	
Organizational Activities	43	National Nursing	
Personal Events	28	Organizations/Activities	19
Work Concerns	24	County and State	
Entertainment	18	Organizations/Activities	9
Trappings and Traditions	4	Community Concerns	10
Total	117	Total	38

Source: Alumnae Association Minutes St. Luke's Training School for Nurses, 1895–1916.

finances, and election of officers. The remaining items, however, were more personal and specific to this particular group of women. These included recognizing marriages and deaths; airing work concerns; planning entertainment; and attending to matters of organizational tradition.

While routine matters such as elections merited little space in the minutes of the organization and provide few insights about the women, descriptions of more personal events fill numerous pages and reveal a great deal about life as a trained nurse. Even the simplest recordings of personal events testify as to what the women considered important. At the "eighth anniversary meeting" of June 1903, for example, special mention was made of the fact that "one of our members married: Miss Wiggins, April 29, 03, class of 1899, to Dr. Judd Goodrich."[17]

Marriage for this organization comprised of young women was indeed a significant event that was regularly highlighted in the group's minutes. Hearty congratulations were extended to a newly married individual, although this expected transition usually meant the loss for a while of an active member. Over time, however, many of those who married resumed their involvement in the association. Thus, as important a change as marriage was to the nurses, even greater import was attached to the permanent loss of a member through death. Numerous expressions of sympathy, for example, followed the death in 1898 of a founding member. Since the woman had little money, a committee was formed "to see how much A Marker [sic] for the grave ... would cost."[18] At the next meeting, the nurses unanimously agreed to use association funds to purchase a gravestone, as homage to their colleague.

Although work issues were raised less often than either organizational matters or announcements of marriage and death, they were distinguished by the intensity of the discussions surrounding them. "Lengthy," "consider-

able," and "warm" is how the nurses described their talks about work matters, while nonwork exchanges evoked no such adjectives. Three issues took
center stage, including a protest of an "unfair hiring decision," needed
improvements for nurses attending to private-duty patients in the hospital, and establishment of a "sick fund."[19] Of these, the sick fund garnered
the most attention.

"After some discussion," which continued late into the evening on
December 4, 1900, the nurses agreed "that we start a fund for sick nurses
belonging to the Alumnae."[20] Although financial support of ill colleagues
was a daunting undertaking, the women were acutely aware of how vulnerable their group was. They received only modest pay and, like most
other workers of this era, they were not protected by health or disability
insurance.[21] As a result, the sick fund became a topic of regular and often
impassioned discourse, much of which centered on maintaining the sol-
vency of the fund.

Their first, rather informal plan was to take "one-quarter of the annual
dues and anyone at any time can add to it."[22] While this proved adequate
for over a decade, the fund was nearly depleted by the summer of 1913. In
an emergency meeting during June of that year, the nurses amended the
rules so that "each member belonging to the sick fund will pay $5.00 annu-
ally." Shortly after, payment became "compulsory for all association members."[23] In an effort to stave off any resistance to these changes, it was also
agreed that the sick fund "be used as a loan fund. No interest to be paid."[24]
Members vigorously endorsed the new plan.

The need to increase revenue was accompanied by a related effort to
more carefully regulate the use of the sick fund. Initially, a nurse who was
seriously ill was eligible for unrestricted assistance. By 1902, however, benefits were limited to "three weeks care . . . special nurses for one week, hospital, (and) drugs."[25] Still, there was never much in reserve and, as a partial
consequence of this fact, members regularly worried about the possible
abuse of the fund by nurses who "might have actually fared well enough on
their own."[26] Thus, the association president eventually appointed a committee "to investigate all cases in need of (the) sick benefit fund . . . and
determine the proper amount to be paid each beneficiary."[27]

Although the committee found no improprieties, the continued payment of members' healthcare expenses ultimately proved to be too great a
burden for the association. St. Luke's was not alone in this regard. Associations across the country were also struggling to meet the medical and nursing needs of their members. Responding to this situation, the National
Nurses' Relief Fund and the Nurses' Sick Benefit Society began offering
health insurance through the American Nurses' Association in 1914.[28]

Once this national plan was in place, the St. Luke's association wasted no time in "discard(ing) the sick fund" later that same year.[29]

With the responsibilities of the sick fund set aside, the nurses turned their attention toward improving the hospital work situation for "special nurses." In actuality, these individuals were far from special, being simply private-duty nurses employed by a private party to look after an individual during hospitalization. Often this meant following a patient from home to hospital and then back home again, because chronic illness, in particular, was seldom resolved by hospitalization. For the patient, this had the advantage of one-to-one, close attention by someone who was familiar with their needs.

Special nurses were not hospital employees, however, and hospital officials tended to overlook their needs. For instance, St. Luke's ignored the requests of individual nurses for "suitable toilet and dressing facilities" in the hospital.[30] Only after the association appointed a committee to "look into this matter," and the group as a whole registered their concern, did hospital officials take steps to remedy the situation. A representative of the hospital board provided written assurance that "facilities for the comfort of the special nurses on duty in the hospital will be made adequate."[31]

Although the issue of toilet and dressing facilities was settled in a relatively amiable manner, members did not shrink from more fervent action when they thought it necessary. For instance, in late 1900 the women unanimously agreed to send a resolution to "the Executive Board of St. Luke's Hospital" protesting the hiring of a graduate from another training school to be in charge of a floor of the hospital. This should not happen, the nurses argued, "when there are (St. Luke's) graduates ready, willing and competent to serve in that capacity."[32] They were adamant in their protest, but the hospital was equally unyielding. The board responded, "There is no precedent on which your Alumnae can base their request." When pressed still further by the nurses, the board president ended discussion with his statement, "We have done in this matter what was deemed best for the Hospital and Training School."[33]

While not always victorious, the nurses proved themselves to have the same strength of will after graduation as had been demanded of them both prior to and during training. These were not shrinking women, to recall the epithet accorded to those who were deemed "too weak" to be nurses. Rather, with a single voice they mobilized their resources to meet the urgent health needs of their members, pushed for work improvements, and showed little hesitation in confronting what they perceived as an unfair work decision.

The women were not solely preoccupied, however, with organizational and work concerns, or in noting passages of marriage and death. They also sought out each other's company for simple enjoyment. Indeed, descriptions of parties and entertainment planning were only slightly less numerous in the minutes than entries focused on work. "Cake and cookies and a social hour" commonly followed the regular meetings.[34] And members helped to plan entertainment for the graduating classes, which included, for example, "a masquerade party, to be held, Monday evening Feb. 15, 1915."[35]

Trappings and traditions, though believed to have been a major preoccupation of early nurses, actually absorbed very little of the nurses' time. Brief entries in the minutes describe the selection of an official class color, badge, and graduate uniform. Members did demonstrate a belief in the importance of their collective efforts by unanimously endorsing a resolution to carefully preserve all of the association's records.[36] Such planning with an eye to the future—the long-term future—strongly suggests a group of people aware of the larger world and their place in it.

Critics of hospital training might see the graduates' focus on "home hospital" issues as evidence of the formidable obstacles that organized nursing had to overcome on the path to professionalization. As these critics charge, "Fidelity to the 'home hospital,' deeply engrained during training, thwarted efforts to develop broader occupational loyalty."[37] Without a doubt, St. Luke's alumnae paid close attention to nearby issues, such as members' marriages and deaths, the sick fund, fair work practices, and socializing. The potential certainly exists for myopic attention to local concerns of the moment. However, deeper meanings and motivating factors at St. Luke's affirm the coexistence of local as well as broader occupational identities.

As children of the working class, and now skilled workers themselves, the women were following time-honored craft traditions. These traditions emphasized a worker's commitment to mutual aid, burial and commemoration, fellowship and feasting, drama and ceremonial sponsorship.[38] Thus, the nurses established the sick fund for mutual aid. They commemorated important events like marriage and death. They celebrated their fellowship at parties. And they honored the drama and ceremony of nursing through their sponsorship of graduation events and the selection of official symbols and dress.

An important gender consideration is the sense of immediacy in the concerns of nurses, a sense of responsibility to immediate needs. This was possibly more true for nurses than for other working women because caregiving was an expectation in both their home lives and public lives. As important as occupational background was in shaping their concerns, the St. Luke's nurses, like women in general in this period, had been socialized to look after home and family. A "defamilialization" construct offered by current social theorists of gender provides a way of assessing women's autonomy, the division of paid work, and the relationship between paid work and unpaid work.[39] In brief, the negative consequences of women's supposedly innate caregiving tendencies can be seen in their economic dependence on men and their low status in the hierarchy of paid work. For nurses in particular, it seems clear that the combination of caregiving with gainful employment would have constituted a breach of deeply engrained and very visible social norms, were the woman's first identity not recognized to be that of a member of a family. After that (possibly) women could be seen as wage-workers and other kinds of participants in the world outside the home. This construct led more than a few women at St. Luke's to cut short their training in order to attend to sick relatives or to help shore up family finances. Ironically, it might well be the motivation for those women who stayed working in the field to attend to the needs and issues surrounding their home hospital and their occupational group. This study argues that the sense of immediacy associated with women's role in society served to augment nurses' commitment to the needs of the nursing field.

⁓

Nurses' efforts to band together on the county, state, and national levels surged during the late nineteenth and early twentieth centuries. On September 8, 1898, nine nurses, representing the four hospital training schools then in existence in St. Paul, established the first representative association of graduate nurses in Minnesota. They called themselves the Ramsey County Graduate Nurses' Association and "achieved the enviable historic distinction of being the first official registry in the United States established . . . by a representative group of graduate nurses operating without profit and solely for the mutual benefit of the group."[40] This local organization flourished and, forty years later, the membership had grown to twelve hundred.

Elsewhere in Minnesota, other nurses were similarly roused to collective action. In the late summer of 1901, for instance, graduate nurses in neighboring Hennepin County gathered to hear "a paper on the aims and advantages of an organized group, following which the Hennepin County Graduate Nurses' Association was formed."[41] Nurses in Duluth, Mankato, Rochester, and Fergus Falls quickly followed suit, creating four more county associations. Then, in 1905, "a mass meeting . . . brought together about 100 nurses, all full of enthusiasm and ready to organize" on a statewide level. By the end of the meeting, the Minnesota State Graduate Nurses' Association was born, "a society for social enjoyment . . . (nursing) advancement . . . (and) the furtherance of the efficient care of the sick."[42]

Beyond Minnesota, forty-four training school superintendents met at the Chicago World's Fair in June 1893 to establish the first national nursing organization, the American Society of Superintendents of Training Schools (renamed in 1912 the National League for Nursing Education). As they assembled in the Hall of Columbus, these influential nurses heard two divergent messages. The first was from Florence Nightingale who, although not present, sent an address that was read before the entire group. Nightingale wrote, "Nursing proper can be taught only by the patient's bedside and in the sick room or ward . . . it (cannot) be taught by books, though these are valuable accessories if used as such."[43]

Nightingale seems to have had in mind the hundreds of training programs like St. Luke's that extolled the virtue of practical experience and minimized the importance of academics. However, her argument might have been lost on the crowd as it was followed by a different argument from America's most prominent nurse at the time, Isabel Hampton [Isabel Hampton Robb]. Hampton—the first superintendent of the Johns Hopkins Training School—focused on educational standards for nurses. She highlighted calls for the standardization of teaching methods, for adding an additional year of training, and for emphasizing theory in nursing education. Other nursing leaders, including Lavinia Dock and Louise Darche, echoed Robb's message.[44] As discussed earlier in this chapter, this particular world's fair in 1893 set a tone at least within the United States for corporate organizational structure. It is understandable that in such a context nurses, too, in establishing their new organization, would adopt the top-down, hierarchical model of efficiency put forward by business leaders.

Symbolic of an ideological divide in nursing, the superintendents' society formed as an elite group to which members were selected according to "the standing of the school over which the candidate presided." It never considered expanding its membership to include the great majority of nurses.[45] Instead, the superintendents' organization suggested the formation of another organization for the rank-and-file—one comprised of alumnae group members. Therefore, following an 1896 meeting of delegates from alumnae associations across North America, the Nurses' Associated Alumnae of the United States and Canada (later the American Nurses Association) was established.

St. Luke's graduates embraced the larger movement to unite nurses; in the sixty alumnae meetings sampled for this study, ideas for ways to aid national nursing efforts came up nineteen times-in almost a third of all meetings. For instance, the president of the group in June 1900 "spoke about our joining the Associate Alumnae" and members expressed their complete support. Without hesitation, or any of the "warm discussions" that marked the controversial issues, the secretary was immediately instructed "to write and find out how we would go about it."[46] A short time later, it was noted that "we have been accepted in the Nurses' Associated Alumnae . . . our annual fee being $5.00."[47]

Less than a decade after joining this group, the St. Luke's alumnae voted to combine efforts with colleagues across Minnesota "to act as hostess to the graduate nurses of the country."[48] They were determined to hold a major convention in the summer of 1909 that would bring together members of both the Nurses' Associated Alumnae and the American Society of Superintendents. This was a daring plan for nurses who had organized on a statewide basis only four years earlier. It demonstrated a bold sense of occupational identity at the national level. Probably because of the nature of sexual politics at the time, the nurses' intrepid organizing efforts were trivialized in the local press, reported under the headline "Nurses Plan a Week of Gaiety."[49]

The impression of unity given by the press was equally misleading. When the convention actually got underway on June 9, 1909, the group was divided literally as well as ideologically. Rather than hold joint meetings, the superintendents met separately in St. Paul while the alumnae group convened its own gathering across the Mississippi River in Minneapolis. The two groups were separated by more than a river, though.

Elevated in economic standing and social status ("bearing the stamp of gentility"), members of the superintendent's society were an elite even among superintendents, since admission into this group was based on the prestige of the program that they supervised.[50] Being the head of a program like St. Luke's, for example, while it ensured respectability, did not merit an invitation to join the society. The superintendents continued to use their organization to push for standardization of training and greater emphasis on theory in nursing. In contrast, the alumnae association represented thousands of nurses, most of whom were employed in private duty.[51] Like the women of St. Luke's, they were working-class individuals who were focused on concerns about adequate jobs, fair pay, and health insurance, rather than intellectual standards.

Although the convention did nothing to bridge the gap between these two groups, it was still considered "a grand success" in bringing so many nurses to the state. At its end, graduates from St. Luke's and similar programs throughout North America took with them much more than the official souvenirs, which included "a miniature hot-water bag with the

Minnesota gopher stamped on the side and a post-card of real birch bark."[52] They left with a deep and enduring sense of the larger nursing community and their place in it.

For the St. Luke's alumnae, the convention experience reinforced their ties to other nurses. This was reflected in their continued interest in national activities and organizations, ranging from sending a delegate to each succeeding convention of the national association, to announcing that "the reports of the Third International Congress of Nurses have been received and are at the Club House—they are worth reading."[53] The women maintained a similar interest in nursing at the state and county levels. For instance, "a copy of the report of the special committee of State Assc.[sic] was read" to the members at a January 1914 meeting, after which the women voted to increase their yearly dues to $2.50, "fifty (cents) of which was to be paid to State Assc."[54] Moreover, in 1916, the group gave their written support to a county-level decision to move the "place of assembly for the Ramsey Co. Registered Nurses' Association from the present one, on Cedar Street, to a more central and easily excessive[sic]."[55]

The nurses maintained a broader occupational focus in their involvement with other matters as well. Despite the contentious environment surrounding early-twentieth-century discussions of family planning, for example, alumnae members sponsored "a talk by Mrs. Margaret Sanger on birth rate control."[56] They sent announcements of the event to women throughout the Twin Cities, encouraging them to come to St. Luke's to hear this controversial and internationally known crusader. In addition, the nurses lent their time and money to aid the Associated Charities of Minnesota, to provide disaster relief to victims of floods and fire, to promote the activities of the Red Cross, and to support the establishment of a memorial fund in honor of the Johns Hopkins nursing leader, Isabel Hampton Robb.[57]

Far from being a self-absorbed or insular community, the women of St. Luke's consistently affirmed their ties to other nurses. Moreover, they did this from the earliest years of the program and during a period in which all of organized nursing was in its infancy.[58] Of course, evidence of a larger occupational consciousness was certainly not a unique occurrence among women workers. The nurses were acting in accord with women in other jobs who, during the early 1900s, "forged alliances" and built "collective identities," efforts that culminated in the development of organizations such as the International Ladies Garment Workers Union and the Women's Trade Union League.[59] Nurses, like increasing numbers of women in the United States, had an identity based on their occupation. What was unique about nursing, however, was the profound separation between average nurses and the field's leaders. While this did not prevent graduates from identifying with a larger nursing community, the gap absorbed nurses' energies and frustrated their attempts at unionizing, as it must have slowed and frustrated the nursing elite in their efforts at professionalization.[60] Indeed, nurses had to wait until November 1973 for national leaders to finally agree to "a campaign . . . to organize RNs" for collective bargaining.[61] The clash in nursing doomed the possibility of a union for decades and it thwarted efforts to unite nurses behind a single occupational ideal.

To this point, we have concentrated on the words of the St. Luke's alumnae. Their silences are as important as their words in understanding the difference between their view of nursing and that of the field's elite. For example, terms that filled the rhetoric of prominent nurses, such as "profession" and "professional," were noticeably absent from the dialogue of the St. Luke's nurses. Neither term occurs in any of the alumnae association's earliest documents, including the articles of incorporation, though the terms appeared constantly in the writings of the nursing elite. Not once were these terms mentioned in the association's minutes. Clearly for this group of women the words "nursing" and "profession" were not used in the same sentence.

The alumnae records are equally silent on the professionalization issues of "educational reform" and "standardization." Though these were key items on the agenda of nursing leaders, the women of St. Luke's failed to make a single reference to either issue. In fact, the very word "education" is absent from their records. They clung instead to the term "training." Moreover, even in using this term, and in discussing their school, the St. Luke's graduates left no record of any conversation about training reform. Nor did they once refer to other topics of pressing interest to the leadership, such as licensure and autonomy.

To read this silence as a repudiation of a larger nursing community would be going too far, however. While silent on professionalization, the St. Luke's nurses were unfailing in their recognition of colleagues at the national, state, and county levels. In contrast, a historian of early-twentieth-century Philadelphia nursing argues that "a dichotomy between (alumnae) members' personal and professional interests," along with "the additional conflict regarding institutional loyalty," ultimately led graduates in that city to resist participating in the larger nursing community.[62] The findings from St. Luke's suggest, however, that nurses in Philadelphia might have been resisting only the professional plans of nursing leaders.

Still, those who tend to see nursing history as an unfolding process of professionalization might interpret the silences as forced upon the women by a paternalistic system of training and work that put professional goals outside the reach of most nurses. Another interpretation might be that, while oppression based on gender certainly influenced various aspects of nursing, this does not completely explain the nurses' behavior. In reality, nurses were active participants in their apprenticeship system of work and training. Despite its faults, this system was viewed as offering positive work opportunities; it led women into a hybrid life that combined the essence of appropriate gender-norm interest with wage-earning ability and occupational solidarity.[63] Abandoning this system in favor of the more academic, university-based model adopted by medicine—the enduring hope of nursing's elite—was completely outside most nurses' frame of reference, at least at St. Luke's. Therefore, the women were quiet in regard to calls for professional reforms, favoring dialogue instead on the more immediate issues relevant to the apprenticeship culture of nursing, such as fair work practices.

Steadfast and Skilled

Training to be a nurse was definitely not an easy path in the St. Luke's era, anymore than it is today. Still, hospital programs offered considerable security, providing the company of others engaged in the same endeavor, basic health care, a place to live, food to eat, a small salary, and the chance to learn skills perceived as lasting a lifetime. Once a woman graduated and closed the doors of the nurses' residence behind her for the last time, these assurances disappeared and she was met full force by the uncertainties of life as a trained nurse. "Instead of feeling elated when her hard-earned diploma was placed in her hand," one Twin Cities nurse explained about her colleagues, "she was more likely to be filled with anxiety for the future."[64]

If the nurse were like the vast majority of graduates across the country, her first task was to find work in private duty. "Except for the few hospital positions, 'nursing' meant private duty," until supplanted by institutional nursing in the 1940s.[65] Here the nurse would need to call upon all of the pragmatism and forcefulness of her training, if she were to be successful in her new, freelance role. "She was thrown entirely on her own resources, unaided by organization or precedent," an independent contractor, negotiating directly with physicians, patients, and families regarding pay and work expectations.[66] Her fortunes as a nurse would rise or fall on the basis of what others said about her abilities in the sick room. Small wonder, then, that everyday work issues dominated meetings of the St. Luke's alumnae.

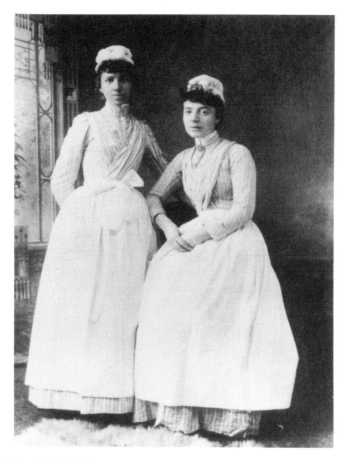

Figure 10. Two St. Luke's Nurses, ca. 1890. From Minnesota Historical Society's Collection #143.B.20.4(B), Box 8, United Hospital Records, Folder: Group photos, ca. 1900–1979.

Still, according to a Department of Labor investigation, nurses who did secure work were paid well in comparison to women in other occupations. Turn-of-the-century weekly wages for women outside of nursing ranged from a high of $6.91 in San Francisco to a low of $3.93 in Richmond.[67] In contrast, private-duty nurses in Minnesota received $15 to $30 per week.[68] An article in the *New York Tribune,* in 1890, proclaimed "trained nurses receive good pay in comparison with that of the ordinary employments of women, ranging from ten dollars per week upward to twenty, thirty or even forty dollars, according to the difficulty of the case."[69] What the newspaper article failed to point out, however, was that like most freelance work nursing tended to be episodic, marked by overwork for some months and idle-

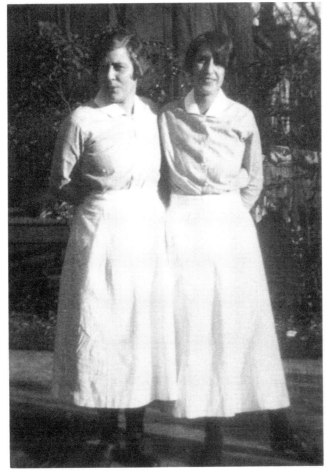

Figure 11. Two St. Luke's Nurses, 1926. From the authors' personal collection.

ness during others.[70] In addition, like other independent practitioners in business for themselves, nurses sometimes found that they could not collect their fees.

The particular uncertainty of private-duty nursing is reinforced by the common experience of regular geographic and job mobility for St. Luke's graduates. In one example, a woman practiced nursing for seven years after completing training in 1914. During this period she found work first in New York City, then served with the Red Cross in South Carolina during World War I, and finally took up nursing in Connecticut. Interspersed with these moves, she spent two summers with her family in La Moure, North Dakota, doing private duty.[71] For another nurse, who graduated in 1926, six years of nursing brought work in St. Paul, Minneapolis, parts of rural Minnesota, and San Francisco.[72] According to the alumnae records, both individuals left paid nursing to get married.

The women responded to the precariousness of their situation by drawing upon and solidifying bonds of friendship established in training (see figures 10 and 11). "Oh yes," a 1906 graduate of neighboring Luther Hospital remarked, "some of the dearest friends I've had were those friends that I was together with while in training."[73] Although this nurse was fortunate in that her initial job away from the hospital "paid me in advance because they knew I was hard up I suppose," she soon had to look for employment elsewhere.[74] Her first case had lasted just three weeks. She now turned for help to a friend from training, a woman "a year older than I (who) was nursing in North Dakota." Taking leave from her own responsibilities, the friend "came to St. Paul and said, 'You've just got to come back with me to Minot, North Dakota.' So I did. I did private duty up there . . . it was all private duty."[75]

Close relationships had other practical advantages as well. As one Minneapolis nurse reflected of her work in the early 1900s, "The private duty nurse of that day will tell you that telephones were not as common then as they are today, nor were they considered as absolutely necessary. Frequently the nearest telephone was at the corner drug store where arrangements were made for the delivery of messages. Several nurses often roomed in the same house and received their calls in common, which obviously made it more convenient. . . ."[76] Yet the importance of friendships from training extended well beyond the bounds of convenience.

Many nurses continued to live and work together long after they left the hospital. For instance, when Elise Rasmus and Phyllis Dudrey completed training at St. Luke's, in October 1933, they left together for work in a hospital in Shreveport, Louisiana. The superintendent of the Shreveport hospital was Miss Dudrey's sister. In a fond letter to the nursing superintendent at St. Luke's, Miss Dudrey described their trip south: "We had a perfectly lovely trip. . . . I think we made a record at the same time. I guess it really is nothing to boast about, but still—we made the distance from Des Moines, Ia., to Little Rock, Ark. in a day's jaunt. You see there are no especially nice hotels anyplace between those cities and each has a lovely one. Miss Rasmus joins me in sending best regards."[77]

The Dudrey sisters and friend worked together for several years in Louisiana before all three moved, in 1941, to Lexington, Kentucky. Another letter, this time from Miss Rasmus, conveyed her affection and also explained the move:

How is everything at St. Luke's? I trust you are well and have as much "fight" as ever. . . . (We) came to Kentucky last summer to work . . . Miss Lucile Dudrey, Phyllis' sister, is Superintendent here, and as we had worked together in Shreveport, Louisiana, for a number of years, she asked me to come to Lexington. . . . This is a 20 bed Unit but we have a hard time keeping within that number, often we run over. Am enjoying Kentucky a lot, the scenery is beautiful—the horse farms are just huge estates set in gorgeous setting. . . . Do hope you will come to Lexington and we can show you some of the beauties of the state.[78]

According to the alumnae records, Miss Rasmus left Kentucky during the mid-1940s and was married. No further information was listed about the Dudreys.

For two other St. Luke's nurses, close ties from training kept them together throughout their work in nursing and into a second occupation. When both completed training, in 1915, they moved to the same address on a busy St. Paul street and began private-duty nursing. In 1917, the women left private duty and enlisted in the Army Nurse Corps, serving alongside one another in Texas and France. After the war, they returned to St. Paul, once again taking up a common residence. Then, apparently disenchanted with nursing, the two embarked on new careers as stenographers. The alumnae records continued to list the women as living together as late as 1940.[79]

Such close relationships between women were openly acknowledged, although the possibility that involvements at times grew into romance drew only whispers.[80] When lifelong companions Etta Paul and Louise Kellogg, registrar and assistant registrars of the neighboring Hennepin County Graduate Nurses' registry, decided in June 1925 to resign, colleagues and friends expressed "profound regret (about) their going." Sorrow was assuaged, however, by the accompanying announcement that "Miss Paul and Miss Kellogg . . . have a home in Carmel-by-the-Sea, California, which they declare to be the most beautiful place on earth and to which they both plan to retire."[81]

Aside from the more personal benefits of companionship, however, the close relationships forged in training undoubtedly helped to sustain the women as they endured the formidable demands of their job. Private-duty nursing was unquestionably strenuous work, often requiring weeks of continuous service, twenty-four hours a day. Yet the women never mentioned this fact in the written records that they left. When asked in the interviews about the rigors of private duty, the nurses simply repeated that long hours and hard work were "to be expected."[82] Still, the women left no doubt about the importance of their connections to fellow trainees and graduates, something that made them more alike than different from other women in the workforce.

Devoted friendships among working women had emerged as a regular topic of popular literature as early as the mid-nineteenth century. In a society where the dominant ideology of separate gender spheres rigidly cast paid employment as the prerogative of men, women workers were "forced by circumstances to create a world unto themselves"; in this world, their relationships were crucial to "sustaining them through their difficult and good times."[83] For most of the nurses, however, the bonds of friendship ultimately loosened and paid work in nursing was set aside to make way for marriage and family.

∾

"I hope you will complete this form so I can do part time nursing again," wrote a St. Luke's graduate to the superintendent of nurses.[84] The nurse's letter was sent in April 1958, twenty-five years after she had completed training. As she noted, "I haven't done any nursing for years, not since I was married but now my children are grown and I have a personal interest because Mom is a patient in a Nursing Home here and they are so short of help and I decided that would be a fine place to work."[85] A few weeks later, a classmate of this nurse wrote to the same superintendent requesting information to complete "an application blank for license as a registered nurse for the state of North Dakota." The woman explained, "As I was married shortly after my graduation I never bothered applying for my license, but am now a widow and would like very much to be back into nursing."[86]

Similar messages were sent year after year by numerous other graduates. Each noted that she had worked for several years after training, then left paid nursing to marry and raise a family, "natural ends" that were thought to be incompatible with employment outside the home.[87] Decades later, and with children grown and often facing other major family changes as well, many sought to return to the nursing workforce. This career pattern, which was confirmed by statistical analysis of nursing employment nationally, reflected not only the tangible obstacles to combining work such as private duty with marriage, but also the values and expectations of the larger society.[88] These values and expectations were echoed in countless subtle and not-so-subtle ways during the late nineteenth and early twentieth centuries. For instance, one St. Luke's superintendent of nursing summarized her evaluation of a first-year nurse with this high praise: "She would be charming in a home of her own."[89] Charm was not a criterion for successful nursing but in this context the term is clearly gendered and illustrates the congruence that nurses valued between their homes lives and their work lives. Expectations were that a job was not a life but family created the context for a life, therefore family took precedence over paid work. Women were not entitled to make this choice for themselves, however; it was a given—and a woman's lifetime was taken.

The recursive relationship between work and home trapped nursing in a low status relative to medicine. With a high turnover and the loss of the energy of young practitioners, nursing was not in a position to compete with medicine for status, money, or authority. Ironically, in the theoretical debates of the 1980s, an opposite argument was based on a similar proposition. The notion that women share a special nature or identity centered on caring and nurturing backed calls for an end to the ghettoization of women in the home and for the feminization of the public domain, which would benefit from the introduction of women's unique characteristics. For the women of St. Luke's, however, in the early decades of the twentieth century, gender norms were clear and most women accommodated them willingly.[90]

According to various sources, nurses were not alone in leaving employment when it conflicted with "their primary means of identification," marriage and family.[91] Women's commitment to family values was the reason for their short-term participation in paid employment, explains one expert on women and work.[92] As a result, two feminist historians note, women moved between domestic and paid labor in response to family needs.[93] For the women of St. Luke's, the combination of marriage and paid nursing was not even considered an option. "I will attend my husband, be his nurse, diet his sickness, for it is my office, and will have no attorney but myself," is the revealing verse that was tucked in the personal papers of a St. Luke's nurse who left private duty to become married.[94] Hence, in the records that the hospital and the alumnae group kept of graduates after training, women were listed as private-duty nurse, institutional nurse, *or* married. None were ever listed as married *and* employed in nursing.[95]

A small percentage of nurses challenged societal trends by never marrying and, instead, staying in paid nursing. One such individual, Irene Dillon, completed her training at St. Luke's in 1900 and found steady employment in nursing for more than thirty years. Her career, as recorded by the alumnae association, typified the geographic and job mobility of nurses, although it was somewhat unique in terms of the number of institutional positions filled:

· 1900 to 1901, Private duty nursing in St. Paul.
· 1901 to 1902, Assistant to the superintendent "in the office" at St.Luke's.
· 1903 to 1904, Private duty nursing in St. Paul.
· 1905 to 1906, Assistant superintendent at St. Luke's.
· 1906 to 1907, Abroad with a patient.
· 1908 to 1911, Private duty nursing in St. Paul.
· 1912 to 1913, Chief nurse at Homestake Hospital in Lead, South Dakota.
· 1914 to 1919, Superintendent at Mandan Hospital in Mandan, South Dakota.
· 1920 to 1921, Superintendent at Pasadena Hospital, Pasadena, California.
· 1921 to 1922, Superintendent at Paulina Stearns Hospital, Ludington, Michigan.
· 1922 to 1925, Superintendent at Lakeview Memorial Hospital, Stillwater, Minnesota.
· 1926 to 1927, Returned to private duty nursing in St. Paul.
· 1927 to 1928, Superintendent at Wichita General Hospital, Wichita Falls, Texas.
· 1928 to 1929, Recuperating following operation in Texas.
· 1930 to (date not given), Private duty nursing (no location given).[96]

Miss Dillon was still unmarried and fifty-four years of age when, for unknown reasons, her work record stopped in 1930.

∿

Whether a woman chose marriage or continued employment in nursing, her identity as a nurse remained unchanged. As Miss Bertsche explained at the start of this chapter, "Once a nurse, always a nurse." Other graduates echoed this theme, emphasizing that there was never a period when they ceased thinking about themselves as a nurse, even though they may have left paid nursing for years at a time. According to one essayist on the craft of nursing, the women's experience and skill had been "absorbed into the banks of memory and the fibers of the nervous system."[97] This was something that could be "called up and counted upon with instant reliability," whether a nurse found herself working in a formal practice setting or her own home.[98]

For the most part, however, historians have been critical of the intermittent employment pattern of early nurses, blaming this pattern for "the difficulty which (nurses) have in committing themselves to a professional career."[99] Recognition of the depth of societal constraints on women's choices in the late nineteenth and early twentieth centuries, however, shifts the blame from nurses to the highly gendered nature of United States society. Observers suggest that, if allowed, nurses would have chosen a career path like that of traditional male professions, devoting themselves to evolving educational standards and a lifelong involvement in the field. However, this suggestion relies less on fact than on the assumption that professionalization is the track followed throughout nursing's history.

In truth, nursing was well suited to the aspirations of women who sought additional opportunities outside the home, while expecting to ultimately focus their energies on marriage and raising a family. In nursing, a woman could acquire specific skills, learn a craft that, as stated at the time, "would be invaluable to her when she embarked on her 'real' roles in life, being a wife and mother."[100] Of course, this was not a new idea or one unique to nursing. "In the name of our sacred family obligations, of the tender services of the mother," nineteenth-century seamstresses were advised, "it is better for women to have a trade than a dowry."[101]

Even as the obstacles to married women working began to crumble, and shorter hours of work made it more feasible to combine family and job, nurses across the country held fast to a pattern of several years' employment after training, then leaving paid nursing for marriage, and finally returning to the workforce later in life.[102] In contrast, women in teaching, who had faced marriage bars similar to nurses yet whose career focus was decidedly more academic gradually changed to a path of uninterrupted employment. In 1910, for example, only 3.6 percent of female teachers were married and working, compared with 7.1 percent of female nurses. By the end of the 1930s, the percentage of female teachers who were married and working had greatly surpassed the corresponding figure for nurses (28.3 percent to 19.0 percent).[103] This change was hastened by the state-by-state imposition in the 1910s of compulsory schooling requirements for children well into adolescence. The increased demand for teachers allowed for the feminization of the formerly male field, and acceptance of married women as teachers also helped end a teacher shortage. Women teachers for their part demonstrated a willingness to persevere in their chosen field despite marriage.

This is not to suggest that average nurses, like those from St. Luke's, lacked loyalty to their chosen field or to other nurses. The women of St. Luke's regularly affirmed their occupational ties, not only locally, but on state and national levels as well. In so doing, they implicitly supported the cause of trained nursing. However, the cause of trained nursing was not the same to them as that of professional nursing. Instead, the nurses' viewpoints and concerns exemplified those expressed by generations of skilled craftsmen, with the exception of different reproductive roles that had to be accommodated. Still, as we'll see in the final chapter, the nature of nursing for these women was far more than a restatement of another male-identified model.

8

Reclaiming the Past, Remaking the Future

Today we are living at the close of one era and at the beginning
of another. . . . The inexorable drive of progress brings us face to
face with needed adjustments, newer methods, newer visions,
and wider hopes. The best of the old era must be retained, the
best of the new adopted.
—Janet Geister, 1931, *The Minnesota Registered Nurse*[1]

After the last woman who had been admitted to the St. Luke's program finished her training on June 20, 1937, the school closed. No
formal observances or fanfare marked the event. After all, the
school was respected, but not great. Even in closing, St. Luke's was just part
of local and national trends. Between 1930 and 1935, the number of hospital schools of nursing in Minnesota plummeted from fifty-one to thirty-
six, likely prompting more than one nurse who read Geister's statement
above to wonder if this was really progress.[2] Outside the state, the situation
was the same, with the number of accredited schools declining nationally
from 2,286 in 1929 to 1,472 in 1936.[3]

No doubt many women were rueful over these changes, since access to
training was becoming increasingly limited. Nursing leaders, however,
regarded the closings as a much-needed step in making way for collegiate
education in nursing. Yet to their disappointment, the number of programs associated with colleges increased to only seventy in the mid-1930s,
nearly all of which represented two years of general education either before
or after a conventional three-year hospital training program.[4]

"With regard to discontinuing our training school at St. Luke's Hospital," the nursing superintendent wrote to the parent of an applicant, "it was
done primarily because we felt that greater opportunities awaited our

143

entering group at the University Hospitals."[5] This was, however, merely an attempt to put a more positive face on the school's dissolution. As the superintendent later explained in a letter to the New York Board of Nurse Examiners, "We have found it unadvisable to enter a class . . . the oversupply of nurses in this locality was becoming a grave problem for a while and we decided to staff with graduates for the time being."[6]

"For the time being" became permanent, as the national economic depression of the 1930s deepened and fewer patients were able to afford private duty. Hospitals responded by permitting more graduates to remain at work, often providing only a small increase in wages over what they had received as students. With the turn away from a staff of apprentice nurses, the number of fully trained nurses in hospitals across the country rose an astounding 700 percent in less than ten years, from four thousand in 1929 to twenty-eight thousand in 1937 (the last year of the St. Luke's school).[7] Obviously, many other hospitals besides St. Luke's rethought the need for a nursing school in this period. The Great Depression alone was not enough to account for so many program closings, however, some of which were in hospitals that were highly solvent and boasted a long and satisfying tradition of nurses' training.

"Tradition . . . (was) the major reason why some of those hospitals that had schools . . . were so reluctant to either improve it or decided to discontinue it," offered a prominent member of the Minnesota Board of Nurse Examiners and a former president of the Minnesota Nurses Association.[8] This individual was speaking in regard to the increased attention that the board was giving to enhancing academics in nursing schools during the early 1930s, and her comment could not have rung more true for St. Luke's. Similar to hospital and school officials across the country, those at St. Luke's diligently complied with board suggestions regarding practical training, while altogether ignoring recommendations for improvements in classroom education.[9] Every action that they took in guiding training at the hospital articulated Nightingale's contention that nursing was "impossible to learn from any book."[10] After more than forty years of this singular vision of nursing, they were not about to abandon it and retool themselves and their program for an academic ideal touted by a relatively small but increasingly influential nursing elite. Nor could they continue indefinitely to subvert the new agenda while purporting to accommodate it. Thus, closing was the most reasonable alternative.

~

For the women of St. Luke's, widespread economic despair and ominous clouds of war in Europe and Asia provided a dishearteningly fitting backdrop to a long-established system of training and work that surely felt under siege, both from forces within and outside nursing. The mainstay of their employment—private duty—was rapidly disappearing, along with many of their schools, while arguments for a type of professionalization that put academics at center stage were being made more forcefully than ever. Uncertainty must have seemed to lurk in every corner, a situation that has parallels to modern nursing. "We are a profession under fire," advise the current editors of the *American Nurse*. They further caution, "Threats to both nursing practice and the profession itself are on the upswing."[11]

Little seems to have changed in the underlying nature of the threats, despite the passage of time and a steady stream of technological miracles within nursing and medicine. Now, as in the past, nursing is assailed by cost-containment pressures, changing work expectations, a lack of clarity about what nursing is and what nurses do, and a resulting void in which "nurses nationwide are finding themselves replaced by technicians and care assistants."[12] Nursing leaders have responded predictably, echoing past calls for nurses to identify their unique contributions to the field of health and to unite behind the vision of nursing reflected in these contributions. Nursing's "salvation . . . must be built on a unity of purpose and a shared vision," insists one such individual, who begins her argument with the desperate question, "Does nursing have a future?"[13]

Of course nursing has a future, but it might or might not be built on the efforts or ideas of those who are themselves nurses today. Whether one defines nursing as "handling, managing and controlling," or as "caring," the face-to-face, hands-on work of nursing is increasingly being given over to individuals who lack the legal title of nurse, but who regularly tend to the needs of patients.[14] At the same time, those who possess the title find themselves positioned farther and farther from the bedside. This is not happening because nursing has been overpowered by medicine, or because of a tightening national budget, although these are important forces with which nursing must contend. It is happening because of the profound lack of appreciation of both of the field's disparate traditions—craft and profession. Recognizing and embracing the whole of nursing's past is likely the key to its most coherent possible future.

In the absence of this appreciation, academic and craft traditions will continue to collide and urgent calls for unity will be repeated again and again, without success. Meanwhile, workplace decisions about nursing will remain in the hands of non-nurses, chief among them health administrators, physicians, and insurance executives. To be sure, the largest of the health occupations would wield an awesome power, if nurses could come together behind a shared vision, a reconceptualization of what nursing is about. To begin with, nurses could finally end debate on the contentious issue of basic entry into practice, bringing some clarity to a confusing situation in which individuals may become registered nurses with a two-year community college degree, a hospital diploma, or a four-year baccalaureate degree.[15]

With entry into practice decided, nurses would then have some credibility in explaining to government and hospital officials, as well as to the general public, just what are the requirements for safe and competent nursing. But entry into practice is no more than the opening scene of a lengthy drama that has gripped nursing in the United States for over a century. At the heart of this drama is the still unanswered question, "What is nursing?" "We must decide who and what is a nurse," one nurse aptly decrees, if we are to stem "our tribalism."[16] Indeed, this is "the taunting question," as another observer points out, which has plagued nursing "throughout its existence."[17] Without a clear answer, unity will remain elusive.

The women of St. Luke's, witness this account, had little uncertainty about the nature of nursing. Nurses did the work of nursing, which consisted of handling, managing, and controlling individuals and situations in health-related settings, with the goal of producing neat, finished-appearing work. Far more than being mere words, this describes how the women of St. Luke's lived in every part of their work and training. It was the underlying message, understood by applicants and their supporters, that this was a field that demanded practical knowledge, physical strength, and emotional stamina. In training, this understanding of nurses and nursing determined that "shrinking, timid women" would not succeed. The same was true after training as well, in a field in which nearly all practitioners during the period of study were essentially independent contractors. The trained nurse was aware of these traits and apparently considered that she maintained them, whether or not she was gainfully employed in nursing at every point in her adult life.

The majority of nurses today, made up primarily of hospital and community college graduates, are heirs to the tradition of nursing epitomized at St. Luke's. Although few practice with the independence of their forebears, they continue to express very similar ideals. "When the private duty nurse left her independent role to become a general duty 'floor' nurse, she left behind her one-to-one relationship with the patient, plus the autonomy and creativity" of her past, states one historian, though she held firmly to a belief in the importance of inner "toughness and determination" while continuing to prize "experience and practical learning above all else."[18] Academia and academics, on the other hand, remained a source of suspicion and disdain as a perceived threat to the real work (i.e., craft) of nursing.

So ingrained are these ideas that most nurses would simply say, "This is nursing," while few would realize that their definition is based on a more than one-hundred-year-old craft tradition that is unique to this field. Despite their unawareness, however, their comments provide quick confirmation of the endurance of this tradition. For example, in a recent study of the practitioner's perspective of "the theory-practice relationship in nursing," one nurse was quoted as saying, "You're put out there . . . (with) a very worried, very ill patient and the theory goes out the window. It is experience that will make a good nurse."[19] Another nurse explains, "You know you learn by your mistakes, learn by what you do right and basically from that, like anything they say in a book is fine in theory, but in practice it's different altogether, wildly different in a way."[20]

An even more public reminder of nursing's craft tradition came in a 1980s *Newsweek* editorial in which a nurse at the time, Alice Ream, shared her view that "the art of skilled nursing is . . . dying out," a casualty of the increasing emphasis on academics rather than practical knowledge and skill.[21] In words that could have been written a century earlier, Ream deplored the current situation in which, for example, "wordy pompous dissertations on bacteriology . . . replace skill training in sterile techniques."[22] She adds that such a problem is perpetuated "when some of those nurses who can't measure up in a hospital reach burnout, they return to college, get another degree and become professors of nursing."[23] For the sake of patients and nurses alike, Ream concludes, nurses must return to their roots, ridding themselves of the "bug in their ears about being handmaidens to physicians" and eschewing academia for a "return to skill training."[24]

Similar messages have been replayed over and over in our own experience, including the nurse cited earlier who pointed out that the problem with university nurses is that they take an impressive list of courses but they still "can't control the (hospital) unit."[25] A personal anecdote involves the nurses to whom one of us introduces a new group of baccalaureate students each semester; these nurses are as regular in their polite greetings as they are in observing how unfortunate it is that university students must spend so much time in the classroom and so little time with patients. There are those as well who could scarcely hide their disdain when the same author explained his plan to enter a doctoral program in nursing. As one emphasized, "That is not what nursing is about!"

Yet academics is exactly what nursing is about to those who have picked up the torch of professionalization from nursing's early leaders. For the most part, this remains a relatively small elite, for whom academic credentials still seem the key to solving nursing's abiding crisis of identity. Thus, according to one member of this group, a fellow of the prestigious American Academy of Nursing, the problem in nursing today is that: " . . . there are more than two million nurses, and only 32 percent possess the baccalaureate. This percentage is shocking in a field that has prepared nurses at the college level for almost 100 years and in light of the impressive increase in the number of women undergraduates. The number of nurses who possess graduate preparation is, of course, more appalling—9% have obtained master's degrees, and less than 1% have obtained the doctorate."[26] Oblivious to the historical forces that initiated and perpetuate this situation, this same leader suggests that "maybe it is time to decrease our enrollments and focus on the brightest students, nurturing them to be motivated for *professional* [original emphasis] careers." A related solution, she explains, is "to radically change our educational system to prepare only postbaccalaureate students for professional practice."[27]

This is, in essence, the same stance that nursing leaders have advocated since the first formal courses in nursing were organized. While in the past this meant shunning apprenticeship and focusing on university education, today's leaders tend to ignore the majority of non-university-educated nurses, fastening their sights instead on plans for entry into "professional nursing" at the master's or doctoral level.[28] Nor has the ultimate goal changed—full and unequivocal professional status, equal to that of medicine. Meanwhile, "we might say we are duping the public," as two nurses state in regard to the ongoing confusion surrounding the issue of entry into nursing practice.[29]

Now, as in the era of the St. Luke's nurses, the viewpoint of the leaders would seem likely to elevate a few, leaving behind those who transact the work of nursing. This would widen rather than bridge the ideological chasm between nursing professionals and average nurses. Thus, a university dean of nursing observes that "the distance between the discipline of nursing (i.e., nursing as an academic pursuit) and the practice of nursing is increasing."[30] And an Indiana nurse questions, "With nurses at two million strong, it's inconceivable that we cannot come to a meeting of the minds and demand our place . . . yet we seem unable to get together with one voice."[31] A largely unrecognized and key difficulty, however, is that often nurses have been misled about their past, particularly in regard to traditions that lie at the heart of nursing.

⁓

Nursing's past is not just a record of struggle toward professional status, and to suggest that it is constitutes a narrow view unsupported by the current evidence. That view tends to obscure much of what is unique and real

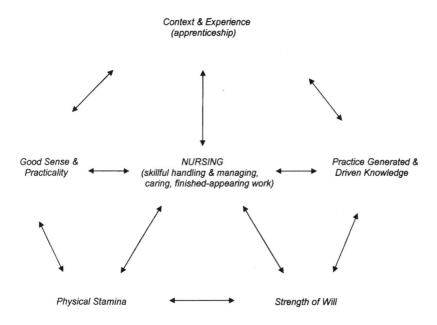

Figure 12. Model of Nursing Adapted from the Women of St. Luke's

about the field. Recognition of this fact is a major legacy of the women of St. Luke's and those represented by their story. In addition, close attention to their story has an importance that extends well beyond the simple recognition of a more complex history. It gives us a chance to rethink our understanding of the nature of nursing, not only in regard to the past, but in terms of the present and future as well. Through this process of revisiting the past and questioning old ideas, we believe it is possible to envision a model of nursing that incorporates and blends the disparate traditions.

The starting point for this new model (see figure 12), as well as for reclaiming nursing's varied history, is understanding that the intense physicality of nursing is a basic characteristic of this field, rather than a symbol of oppression to be overthrown. This characteristic is reflected in the claims of the St. Luke's applicants to a "strong back," the ability to "work and never get tired," and the ability to "walk as many as 12 miles a day."[32] During and after training, the women similarly strove to be "strong and capable in handling patients," realizing that "nursing is a strenuous piece of work even for the most strong."[33] Nor has nursing ceased to be an intensely physical endeavor. For the majority of today's nurses, nursing remains a field that tests the limits of physical endurance, as they monitor, feed, bathe, lift, transfer, and ambulate patient after patient.

This is not to deny the exploitive aspects of nursing experience, either past or present. Rather, it is an acknowledgment of a core reality that defines nursing, a reality that was embraced by the women of St. Luke's and is similarly embraced by contemporary nurses. For some this reality seems to be an embarrassment, as they praise "the exquisite . . . intellectual challenge" of nursing without ever mentioning the equally remarkable physical challenge, except as something to be forsaken.[34] In truth, the physicality of nursing remains a key to understanding the nature of this field and of gender norms, for it continues to defy stereotyped notions of women's fragility.

Just as important as recognizing the centrality of physical stamina in nursing is understanding the importance of a strong will. A woman who lacked "pluck and determination" and had "not much force to her" was as unlikely to succeed in nursing during the era of St. Luke's as she is today. This is contrary to gender-based notions of nursing passivity and saintly submissiveness.[35] Instead, without threatening anyone's femininity, nursing still requires practitioners to be self-reliant, "willing to speak forcefully," and even ready to protest when the situation demands, as occurred when the St. Luke's nurses believed hospital administrators acted unfairly.[36] Indeed, strength of will is implicit to handling, managing, and controlling workers and ward, the definition of nursing at St. Luke's. Despite some of the negative connotations that might surround these terms today (particularly the idea of "controlling") nurses continue to shoulder the major responsibility for ensuring smoothly functioning health settings. Moreover, this responsibility still calls for skillful handling and managing of the physical environment, patients, and personnel. While there certainly are more personnel in nursing contexts now than there were in the period of this study, the need for fully nuanced nursing has not lessened.

The model of nursing that emerges from this narrative, then, is one that acknowledges nursing as an intensely physical undertaking that generally demands of its practitioners both a strong will and a strong body. Also in this model, nursing is seen as something that requires a high level of "good sense and practicality," joined together with the well-honed skills of a craft. "She has a head full of good sense" was a typical description of nursing applicants.[37] During training, women were repeatedly called upon to exercise "real thinking," which was contrasted with a focus on "intellectual concepts."[38] As one nurse was previously quoted as saying, "The practical aspect of nursing . . . must never be sacrificed in the struggle after the more alluring and less substantial adornments," which she equated with academic study.[39]

It was exactly this type of thinking that underlay the solid belief in the importance of apprenticeship training. To be sure, hospital and physician self-interest fed this belief and even used it for exploitive gains, but such self-interest cannot diminish the fact that apprenticeship, as a feature of nursing that predated the first hospital schools, was viewed and continues to be viewed by many nurses as a fundamental element in the process of becoming a nurse. Apprenticeship and nursing may be even more closely linked, as some feminist scholars have argued since the 1980s, by a feminine emphasis on immediacy, meaning hands-on experience and contextual understanding.[40] For women, in this view, knowledge tends to be regarded as "an understanding that needs to be confirmed in context and in use; experience may need to accompany formal expertise . . . there is a need to have knowledge confirmed and validated by others."[41] Unlike classroom learning, which was of minimal importance at St. Luke's, apprenticeship learning was and is rich in terms of context and experience. And this was exactly the type of learning anticipated by prospective nurses, including the 1902 applicant who asked "to enter the hospital in order to complete the instruction and practice" that she had already begun "as assistant to a well-trained and exceptionally good nurse" in her community.[42]

So, too, apprenticeship training seemed to be a fitting expression of the essential qualities of good sense and practicality that nurses were expected to demonstrate. It was consistent also with the overall goal of nursing at St. Luke's—the production of "neat, finished-appearing work." Apprenticeship was the reasonable way of perfecting the craft skills of the nurse, a core feature of nursing, which was epitomized in the twelve steps of bed making, the seventeen steps of giving an injection, and the eighteen steps for administering a hot pack. When all of these related aspects are viewed together—apprenticeship, expectations of good sense and practicality, the goal of finished-appearing work, and the emphasis on craft skill—a closely connected pattern is formed, one that is a crucial part of a unique nursing identity and an equally crucial part of the model being presented here. More than a defense of outmoded traditions in nursing, the lessons from these early nurses also suggest ways to bridge the gap that has so long existed between the leaders of this field and the majority of its practitioners.

The apprenticeship tradition remains a source of power within nursing, though also a source of suspicion when viewed as adverse to purely academic pursuits. Rather than arguing the case of nursing as an exquisite intellectual challenge, or further polarizing the field with calls for entry into practice at the doctoral level, perhaps prominent nurses can carefully tie educational and research goals to the practical needs of patients, as identified by practicing nurses. This will necessarily involve a reaffirmation of the importance of apprenticeship learning in nursing, not as an adjunct to more important classroom teaching, but as an indisputably significant and historically proven key aspect of this field. This need not be a painful step, and indeed might bring some comfort to a field so often split by the sense that it must be either practical or theory-based. In fact, nursing is complete with both elements.

The women of St. Luke's made clear a century ago that conceptualizing nursing as an intellectual endeavor only would widen the divide between nurses. Envisioning the field as comprising practical knowledge and applied skill will help to resolve differences by providing a clear and historically based focus for nurses at all levels. The lack of a common understanding rooted in the realities of nursing practice is evident in the conundrum recently posed by a dean of a university school of nursing, an editor of a scholarly nursing journal. In somewhat self-congratulatory terms, this individual remarked on her admiration of nursing's "stunning successes . . . (and) the clear trajectory" of nursing leaders, then pondered, "I'm less certain if the followers are all aboard the spaceship."[43] The gap between nurses and the leaders in their field, symbolized by the Mississippi River during the 1909 nurses' convention held in Minnesota, is being perpetuated in the twenty-first century.[44] The same lack of agreement on the nature of nursing also fuels a seemingly endless string of contradictory conclusions about nursing's fate, which alternate between dramatic praise—"American nursing has accrued with remarkable speed all the accoutrements of . . . a learned profession"—and dire warnings about the "disintegration of nursing as a distinct profession."[45]

After more than a century of colliding visions, it seems clear that average nurses today are as unlikely as those at the time of St. Luke's to accept an ideal that conflicts with their deeply held beliefs about, and daily experience of, the work of nursing. The story of the women of St. Luke's suggests a way to unite the opposing visions of nursing by grounding the intellectual work of nursing in past and present realities. Physicality, strength of will, an abiding emphasis on practicality, apprenticeship, and a deep pride in craft skills are all essential realities of nursing's past and present. Trying to hide or ignore these realities will only further polarize proponents of the different standpoints on nursing. These ideas can more profitably be blended into a combination of immediate realities and intellectual investigation. Rather than precluding further development of nursing education or research, these two parts clearly indicate the direction that the development of nursing should take.

Nursing education and research, to be appreciated by all nurses, must be driven by practical ends and practicing nurses, rather than the professional inclinations of a relatively small group of leaders. To accomplish this means letting go of the cherished notion that, one day, after sufficient struggle, nursing will finally achieve full professional status, equal to that of medicine. In actuality, the playing field is not level. From roots in a highly gendered time, medicine and nursing developed different bases of power. The gender-specifications of those fields have changed and are changing, but the social power of medicine—in terms of money, status, and organization—is not bending to bring up the "little sister" of nursing to its own level. The harder nursing leaders struggle for all the trappings of a profession, and the more invested they become in the system of hierarchical organization that defines professions, the more likely it is that medicine will increase in stature and nothing will be changed for nursing. Indeed, as one expert on the politics of nursing remarks, "The question we should ask is not 'is nursing a profession?' but 'should nursing want to be a profession.'"[46]

The women of St. Luke's answered this question back when it was first asked by helping to forge a unique occupational model in which sameness with medicine was never an issue. For them, nursing was an entirely separate practice, both in the immediate sense of working with patients and in terms of basic beliefs about the nature of their endeavor. They understood that they were engaged in the most practical of all health occupations, one in which their strength, experience, and skill were prized above all else. It was nursing, not medicine, and as Nightingale once remarked, "woe unto the man" who failed to appreciate the difference.[47] Furthermore, most nurses firmly believed that the key to entering this distinctive field was apprenticeship training.

Apprenticeship was the cornerstone on which rested the entire process of becoming a nurse. It was the route through which trainees came to fully appreciate the comment "Once a nurse, always a nurse." As Melosh remarks,

> For (early) nurses, apprenticeship culture nurtured the intense commitment to work that is more commonly associated with professional training and practice. In oral memoirs, even women who had not been employed for many years continued to identify themselves and to be identified by others as nurses. . . . And most talked wistfully of going back to work someday. Nursing remained a part of them in a way that other women's work simply does not: waitresses, secretaries, teachers, or social workers seldom have such strong and enduring personal and social connections to their work.[48]

This was the unshakable truth that allowed nurses to maintain the highest commitment to their occupation, even amidst a pattern of episodic paid employment shaped by gendered expectations of marriage and family.[49] One does one not have to search widely to find nurses today who chose their career, as one individual recently remarked, in order "to do something that I can believe in, to learn a skill that I'll always have and be able to raise a family."

As compelling as these historic findings might be, however, the challenge that they represent to long-held assumptions of nursing's professionalization track will make them, and the model to which they give rise, difficult for some to accept. Yet reclaiming the entirety of nursing's past opens the way to understanding "not only the exploitative nature of . . . (nursing) work," as one author explains, but to understanding "the positive qualities inherent in it as well as why they seem to get lost when professionalized."[50] With each added piece of information examined, the voices of the women of St. Luke's, recorded in their writings and reports, grow more insistent that we see nurses and nursing not only through the lens of professionalization, but on their own terms and in their own distinct way.

Initially, this seemed to be a direct challenge for this study. Intent on earning our doctorates, we initially set out to join a long list of other writers in exposing the early injustices in this field. Our goal was to complete a paper based on records of the St. Luke's Hospital Training School for Nurses that would defend caring as the historic basis for nursing's claim to special knowledge. The women of St. Luke's, however, turned our preconceptions upside down. Even the near-sacred notion of the tradition of caring in nursing, at least as it is argued by contemporary authors, seems flawed when tested against the real lives of nurses in training.[51] Their description of nursing—handling, managing, and controlling patients, workers, and ward with the aim of producing neat, finished-appearing work—while perhaps constituting caring in a very broad sense, was a different type of tradition than we had expected to observe. Nor were we expecting to see that instead of chafing against such a tradition, nurses embraced it. Their work was not performed as some kind of internalized oppression, but as a tradition to be honored and continued.

In short, our view of nursing's past is clouded when viewed primarily through the lens of professionalization.[52] Recognition of this fact is an important legacy of average nurses, such as the women of St. Luke's. While the programs in which they trained faded away, relatively unnoticed, their real contribution continues on in the form of a unique and enduring approach to nursing, thanks to the availability of the written records the women and the program saved for posterity. Within this approach are the seeds of an alternative model of nursing that can help to remake nursing in the future.

~

The divisions in nursing were already well established when, in 1920, Lavinia Dock and Isabel Stewart made the following observation:

> Every body of workers . . . has its own traditions which have gradually accumulated and which are handed down from generation to generation of new recruits. In this way the whole group is welded together into a more or less homogenous and united body with common aims and a common spirit. Traditions do not, however, always make for progress . . . the best work (of a field) is usually done by building up and strengthening good traditions and institutions and letting the old useless ones die out.[53]

These women, both ardent supporters of professionalization, undoubtedly hoped nursing's craft traditions would fade away. But that did not occur. What has taken place instead is a persistent pattern of renewing the division with every generation of nurses.

The key to stopping this divisive process, as attested to here, lies in recognizing and claiming the traditions of the rank and file as well as the leaders. Gentle hands, expert injections, careful handling of the patient in pain—nursing's craft legacy—must be accorded the same historical legitimacy as the exquisite intellectual challenge of nursing. Only then, as this story of strong and determined women shows, will nurses be able to come together and decide which traditions to strengthen, which to let die, and which to support for the future of nursing.

Notes

Notes to Chapter 1

1. Florence Nightingale, *Notes on Nursing: What It Is and What It Is Not*, 2d ed. (Norwalk, Conn.: Appleton-Century-Crofts, 1860; reprint, New York: Dover Publications, 1969. London: Harrison and Sons, 1860), 8 (page references are to reprint edition).

2. Wendell W. Oderkirk, "'Organize or Perish': The Transformation of Nebraska Nursing Education, 1888–1941" (Ph.D. diss., University of Nebraska, 1988), 7. Also see David G. Allen, "Professionalism, Occupational Segregation by Gender and Control of Nursing," *Women and Politics* 6 (fall 1986): 1–25; and Janet Wilson James, "Writing and Rewriting Nursing History: A Review Essay," *Bulletin of the History of Medicine* 58 (1984): 568.

3. Shiphrah A. Alicia William-Evans and M. Elizabeth Carnegie, "The Evolution of Professional Nursing," in *Contemporary Nursing: Issues, Trends, and Management,* ed. Barbara Cherry and Susan R. Jacob (St. Louis, Mo.: Mosby, 2002), 23. For similar examples see Janice Rider Ellis and Celia Love Hartley, *Nursing in Today's World: Challenges, Issues, and Trends* (Philadelphia: Lippincott, 2001), chap. 5; and Nellie Nelson, "Image of Nursing: Influences of the Present," in *Nursing Today: Transition and Trends,* ed. JoAnn Zerwekh and Jo Carol Claborn (Philadelphia: Saunders, 2000), chap. 3.

4. For a discussion of the pervasive assumption that professions grow through a series of stages called professionalization, see Andrew Abbott, *The System of Professions: An Essay on the Division of Expert Labor* (Chicago: University of Chicago Press, 1988). For an example of how stages of professionalization are applied to nursing, see Nancy Tomes, "'Little World of Our Own': The Pennsylvania Hospital Training School for Nurses, 1895–1907," in *Women and Health in America: Historical Readings,* ed. Judith Walzer Leavitt (Madison: University of Wisconsin Press, 1984), 467–81; Mary Carol Ramos, "The Johns Hopkins Training School for Nurses: A Tale of Vision, Labor, and Futility," *Nursing History Review* 5 (1997): 23–48; or Patricia M. Schwirian, *Professionalization of Nursing: Current Issues and Trends* (Philadelphia: Lippincott, 1998), chap. 1.

5. M. Louise Fitzpatrick, "A Historical Study of Nursing Organization: Doing Historical Research," in *Nursing Research: A Qualitative Perspective,* ed. P. L. Munhall and Carolyn J. Oiler (Norwalk, Conn.: Appleton-Century-Crofts, 1986), 195–96, 223–24.

6. Jane E. Mottus, *New York Nightingales: The Emergence of the Nursing Profession at Bellevue and New York Hospital, 1850–1920* (Ann Arbor, Mich.: UMI Research Press, 1981), 175.

7 Nancy Tomes, "The Silent Battle: Nurse Registration in New York State, 1903–1920," in *Nursing History: New Perspectives, New Possibilities,* ed. Ellen Condliffe

Lagemann (New York: Teachers College Press, 1983), 124–25. A variation on studies such as this one, as well as the examples in the two preceding notes, are histories that are written primarily for celebratory purposes rather than analysis. Numerous training schools, particularly those that evolved into university-based programs, have histories that fit this description. See for example Poldi Tschirch, ed., *A Century of Excellence, A Vision for the Future: The University of Texas School of Nursing at Galveston, 1890–1990* (Galveston: University of Texas Medical Branch, 1990); Margaret Heyse Cory, *Nurse: A Changing Word in a Changing World: The History of the University of North Dakota College of Nursing, 1909–1982* (Grand Forks, N.Dak.: University Press, 1982); and James Gray, *Education for Nursing: A History of the University of Minnesota School* (Minneapolis: University of Minnesota Press, 1960). This genre seems to have had minimal impact on the overall interpretation of nursing history and, as a consequence, is not a focus of this account.

8. Diane Hamilton, "Constructing the Mind of Nursing," *Nursing History Review* 2 (1994): 3–28.

9. The term *occupation* is used in a generic sense to refer to all fields of employment, regardless of other distinctions involved, such as professional, nonprofessional, or trade. A survey of the literature indicates that this is the most neutral term to describe the widest range of employment fields. An exception to this view is presented in Joan E. Lynaugh and Claire M. Fagin, "Nursing Comes of Age," *Image* 20 (winter 1988): 184–90. Lynaugh and Fagin argue that nursing is a profession rather than an occupation.

10. Margarete Sandelowski, *Devices and Desires: Gender, Technology, and American Nursing* (Chapel Hill, N.C.: University of North Carolina Press, 2000), 178–80.

11. Sioban Nelson, *Say Little, Do Much: Nurses, Nuns, and Hospitals in the Nineteenth Century* (Philadelphia: University of Pennsylvania Press, 2001), 152, 156, 160, 164. See also Sioban Nelson, "Entering the Professional Domain: The Making of the Modern Nurse in 17th Century France," *Nursing History Review* 7 (1999): 171–87; and Elaine Sorensen Marshall and Barbra Mann Wall, "Religion, Gender, and Autonomy: A Comparison of Two Religious Women's Groups in Nursing and Hospitals in the Late Nineteenth and Early Twentieth Centuries," *Advances in Nursing Science* 22 (1999): 1–22.

12. Lavinia L. Dock and Isabel Maitland Stewart, *A Short History of Nursing* (New York: G. P. Putnam's Sons, 1920), 347.

13. Mary M. Roberts, *American Nursing: History and Interpretation* (New York: Macmillan, 1954), 201.

14. See, for example, Dock and Stewart, *A Short History;* Roberts, *American Nursing;* Isabel Stewart and Anne S. Austin, *A History of Nursing from Ancient to Modern Times—A World View,* 5th ed. (New York: G. P. Putnam's Sons, 1962); Vern L. Bullough and Bonnie Bullough, *The Emergence of Modern Nursing,* 2d ed. (Toronto: Macmillan, 1969); Josephine A. Dolan, M. Louise Fitzpatrick, and Eleanor Krohn Herrmann, *Nursing in Society: A Historical Perspective,* 15th ed. (Philadelphia: W. B. Saunders Co., 1983); Philip A. Kalisch and Beatrice J. Kalisch, *The Advance of American Nursing,* 3d ed. (Philadelphia: J. B. Lippincott Company, 1995).

15. Oderkirk, *Organize or Perish,* 171, 230.

16. Carolyn Watkins, "The Redefinition of Professional Nursing: The Aultman Hospital School of Nursing Experience" (Ph.D. diss., University of Akron, 1987), iii.

17. Bonnie Ketchum Smola, "A Study of the Development of Diploma and Baccalaureate Degree Nursing Education Programs in Iowa from 1907–1978" (Ph.D. diss., Iowa State University, 1980), 295. Also see Georgia Bernadette von Conrad, "The First Eighty Years: The History of Lutheran Medical Center School of Nursing, 1898–1978" (Ph.D. diss., Saint Louis University, 1980); and Marilyn Givens King, "Conflicting Interests: Professionalization and Apprenticeship in Nursing Education. A Case Study of the Peter Bent Brigham Hospital" (Ph.D. diss., Boston University, 1987). .

18. Ashley, Jo Ann, *Hospitals, Paternalism and the Role of the Nurse* (New York: Teachers College Press, 1976), 18.

19. Susan M. Reverby, *Ordered to Care: The Dilemma of American Nursing, 1850–1945* (Cambridge: Cambridge University Press, 1987), 65, 122.

20. Beatrice J. Kalisch and Philip A. Kalisch, "Slaves, Servants, or Saints? An Analysis of the System of Nurse Training in the United States, 1873–1948," *Nursing Forum* 14 (1975): 225, 232, 251.

21. Linda T. Anglin, "Historical Perspectives: Influences of the Past," in *Nursing Today: Transition and Trends,* ed. JoAnn Zerwekh and Jo Carol Claborn (Philadelphia: Saunders, 2000), 41.

22. Barbara Melosh, "Apprenticeship Culture and Nurses' Resistance to Professionalization," in *Alternative Conceptions of Work and Society: Implications for Professional Nursing,* ed. Carol A. Lindeman (Washington, D.C.: American Association of Colleges of Nursing, 1988), 31–32.

23. Ibid., 34–35.

24. Melosh, "Apprenticeship Culture," 38. Also see Barbara Melosh, *"The Physician's Hand": Work Culture and Conflict in American Nursing* (Philadelphia: Temple University Press, 1982), chap. 1 passim.

25. Sarah T. Colvin, *A Rebel in Thought* (New York: Island Press, 1944), 71.

26. Evelyn Hardy, "Letters," *American Journal of Nursing* 60 (December 1960): 1702.

27. R. Meyer, "Letters," *American Journal of Nursing* 62 (August 1962): 16.

28. Susan Rimby Leighow, "Backrubs vs. Bach: Nursing and the Entry-into-Practice Debate, 1946–1986," *Nursing History Review* 4 (1996): 8–9.

29. JoEllen Koerner, "Differentiated Practice: The Evolution of Professional Nursing," *Journal of Professional Nursing* 8 (November–December 1992): 335; Linda S. Baas, "An Analysis of the Writings of Janet Geister and Mary Roberts Regarding the Problems of Private Nursing," *Journal of Professional Nursing* 8 (May–June 1992): 176; Sam Porter, "The Poverty of Professionalization: A Critical Analysis of Strategies for the Occupational Advancement of Nursing," *Journal of Advanced Nursing* 17 (June 1992): 723.

30. For added insight into the entry-into-practice debate see Janet Wilson James, "Isabel Hampton and the Professionalization of Nursing," in *The Therapeutic Revolution: Essays in the Social History of American Medicine,* ed. M. J. Vogel and C. E. Rosenberg (Philadelphia: University of Pennsylvania Press, 1979), 201–44; American Nurses' Association, *A Case for Baccalaureate Preparation in Nursing* (Kansas City, Mo.: The Association, 1979); Rebecca Partridge, "Education for Entry into Professional Nursing Practice: The Planning of Change," *Journal of Nursing Education* 20 (April 1981): 40–46; M. J. Rajabally, "Point of View: The Entry into Practice Issue, We Have Seen the Enemy," *Canadian Nurse* 78 (February 1982): 40, 42; S. H. Fondiller, "The Entry Issue: How Much Longer? An Historian's View," *Journal of the New York State Nurses Association* 17

(June 1986): 7–14; Margaretta Styles, Sheila Allen, Sara Armstrong, Marsha Matsura, Daphne Stannard, and Julia Stocker Ordway, "Entry: A New Approach," *Nursing Outlook* 39 (September–October 1991): 200–3.

31. Ibid.

32. See, for example, Leighow, "Backrub vs. Bach"; Joan Brady, *Fluff My Pillow, Bend My Straw: The Evolution and Undoing of a Nurse* (Vista Publishing: Long Branch, N.J., 1992); and Anglin, "Historical Perspectives." In discussing the role of colleague, for instance, Anglin rues, "Until nurses can respond to each other with respect, it will be difficult to move from the collaborator to true colleague" (48).

33. Some, such as Colvin, *Rebel in Thought,* have expressed ideas similar to those of Melosh, but none has argued a coherent framework as an alternative to professionalization. See also Margaret Bayldon, "Diploma Schools: The First Century," *RN* 36 (February 1973): 33–48.

34. St. Luke's Hospital Training School Collection, Minnesota Historical Society, St. Paul, Minn. This collection is hereafter cited as SLHTS Collection; Minnesota Historical Society, St. Paul, Minn., is hereafter cited as MHS.

35. See, for example, James, "Isabel Hampton"; Mottus, *New York Nightingales;* Tomes, "'Little World of Our Own'; and King, "Conflicting Interests."

36. St. Luke's Hospital Training School for Nurses folder, Minnesota Board of Nurse Examiners Collection, MHS. This collection is hereafter cited as MBNE Collection.

37. Comparative data to support the overall contention of St. Luke's typicality was also taken from various school files and general discussions, involving both state and national comparisons, in the MBNE Collection. Refer also to the related discussion in chapter 3. The typicality of St. Luke's is also discussed in the following articles: Tom Olson, "Competing Paradigms and the St. Luke's Alumnae Association Minutes, 1895–1916," *Advances in Nursing Science* 12 (June 1990): 53–62; Tom Olson, "The Women of St. Luke's and the Occupational Evolution of Nursing, 1897–1915," *Mid-America, An Historical Review* 73 (April–July 1991): 109–26; Tom Olson, "Laying Claim to Caring: Nursing and the Language of Training," *Nursing Outlook* 41 (March–April 1993): 68–72; Tom Olson, "Apprenticeship and Exploitation: An Analysis of the Work Pattern of Nurses in Training, 1897–1937," *Social Science History* 17 (winter 1993): 559–76; Tom Olson, "Recreating Past Separations and the Employment Pattern of Nurses," *Nursing Outlook,* 43 (September/October 1995), 210–14; Tom Olson, "Balancing Theory and Practice in Nursing Education: Case Study of an Historic Struggle," *Nursing Outlook* 46 (1998): 268–72. For examples of other studies involving nurses' training, see the sources listed in endnote 7 above. For information on the increase in training programs see Wendell W. Oderkirk, "Setting the Record Straight: A Recount of Late Nineteenth-Century Training Schools," *Journal of Nursing History* 1 (November 1985): 30–37; Council on Medical Education and Hospitals of the American Medical Association, "Third Presentation of Hospital Data," *Journal of the American Medical Association* 82 (1924): 118; May Ayres Burgess, *Nurses, Patients, and Pocketbooks: A Study of the Economics of Nursing* (New York: Committee on the Grading of Nursing Schools, 1928).

38. Listing of hospital schools of nursing, 1900–1940, MBNE Collection, MHS; Philip A. Kalisch and Beatrice J. Kalisch, *The Advance of American Nursing,* 3d ed. (Philadelphia: J. B. Lippincott Company, 1995), 312. Refer also to the related discussion in chapter 7.

39. Refer to the previous citation regarding the typicality of St. Luke's. Also see Joan E. Lynaugh, "From Respectable Domesticity to Medical Efficiency: The Changing Kansas City Hospital, 1875–1920," in *The American General Hospital: Communities and Social Contexts,* ed. Diana Elizabeth Long and Janet Golden (Ithaca, N.Y.: Cornell University Press, 1989), 21–39; Paul Starr, *The Social Transformation of Medicine* (New York: Basic Books, 1982), chap. 4.

40. Ellen D. Baer, "The Conflictive Social Ideology of American Nursing: 1893, A Microcosm" (Ph.D. diss., New York University, 1982), 201, 210. Baer reveals her own bias in contrasting preparation for nursing with that "in every other field," since she includes only professional fields in her comparison.

NOTES TO CHAPTER 2

1. Application letters, February 6, 1906 and February 15, 1906, n.d., file "E. Claggett," Box 1, St. Luke's Hospital Training School Collection, Minnesota Historical Society, St. Paul, Minn. This collection is hereafter cited as SLHTS Collection, MHS. Minnesota Historical Society is hereafter cited as MHS.

2. "Annual Report of St. Luke's Hospital," 1892, St. Luke's/United Hospital Collection, Minnesota Historical Society, St. Paul, Minn. This collection is hereafter cited as SL/UH Collection. Instructions to women entering training, ca. 1895, SL/UHC; Nancy Johnston Hall and Mary Bround Smith, *Traditions United: The History of St. Luke's and Charles T. Miller Hospitals and Their Service to St. Paul* (St. Paul, Minn.: United Hospital Foundation, 1987), 24.

3. Hall and Smith, *Traditions United,* 23; Theodore Blegen, *Minnesota: A History of the State* (Minneapolis: University of Minnesota Press, 1975), 448–53; Virginia Brainard Kunz, *Saint Paul: The First 150 Years* (St. Paul, Minn.: Saint Paul Foundation, 1991), 47–48.

4. "Minutes of the Board of Trustees," 1883, SL/UH Collection, MHS.

5. "Annual Reports of St. Luke's Hospital," 1881, 1883, 1887, SL/UH Collection, MHS.

6. St. Luke's was not alone in seeking to attract patients. As Lynaugh explains, "The explosive growth of hospitals after the Civil War was a social response to care demands from city dwellers, many of whom were willing to pay for care" (Joan E. Lynaugh, "Narrow Passageways: Nurses and Physicians in Conflict and Concert Since 1875," in *The Physician as Captain of the Ship: A Critical Reappraisal,* ed. Nancy M. P. King, Larry R. Churchill, and Alan W. Cross [Boston: D. Reidel Publishing, 1988], 23).

7. "Annual Report of St. Luke's Hospital," 1889, SL/UH Collection, MHS.

8. Kunz, *Saint Paul,* 46–48; June Drenning Holmquist, ed., *They Chose Minnesota: A Survey of the State's Ethnic Groups* (St. Paul: Minnesota Historical Society Press, 1981), 1–14.

9. Stanton A. Glantz, *Primer of Biostatistics* (New York: McGraw-Hill, 1992), 1–2.

10. "Annual Report of St. Luke's Hospital," 1894, SL/UH Collection, MHS.

11. "Annual Reports of St. Luke's Hospital," 1892, 1894, SL/UH Collection, MHS. Also see Hall and Smith, *Traditions United,* 27.

12. For a discussion of the uncertain state of medicine during this era see Kenneth M. Ludmerer, *Learning to Heal: The Development of American Medical Education*

(Baltimore, Md.: Johns Hopkins University Press, 1995); Kenneth M. Ludmerer, *Time to Heal: American Medical Education from the Turn of the Century to the Era of Managed Care* (New York: Oxford University Press, 1999); Thomas Neville Bonnner, *Iconoclast: Abraham Flexner and a Life in Learning* (Baltimore, Md.: Johns Hopkins University Press, 2002).

13. Paul Starr, *The Social Transformation of Medicine* (New York: Basic Books, 1982), 95–100. For further discussion of homeopathy and allopathy see Harris L. Coulter, *Divided Legacy: The Conflict Between Homeopathy and the American Medical Association: Science and Ethics in American Medicine, 1800–1900,* vol. 3, 2d ed. (Berkeley: North Atlantic Press, 1988); Naomi Rogers, *An Alternative Path: The Making and Remaking of Hahnemann Medical College and Hospital of Philadelphia* (Rutgers: Rutgers University Press, 1998); and Martin Kaufman, *Homeopathy in America: The Rise and Fall of a Medical Heresy* (Baltimore, Md.: Johns Hopkins Press, 1971).

14. "Minutes of the Officers and Trustees," 1891–1902, SL/UH Collection, MHS.

15. "Homeopathy and Allopathy Debate," 1881–1901, SL/UH Collection, MHS. Also see Hall and Smith, *Traditions United,* 28.

16. "Minutes of Staff Meetings," 1900–1906, SL/UH Collection, MHS; "Minutes of the Officers and Trustees," 1891–1902, SL/UH Collection, MHS.

17. "Minutes of the Officers and Trustees," 1901, SL/UH Collection, MHS.

18. "Minutes of the Officers and Visitors," 1897–1902, SL/UH Collection, MHS. Also see Hall and Smith, *Traditions United,* 33.

19. Kalisch and Kalisch, *Advance of Nursing,* 107–8. The proliferation of training schools, in the wake of a similar increase in hospitals, highlights the schools' importance. Indeed, the opening of the St. Luke's Hospital Training School for Nurses was part of a nationwide increase in training programs, from 16 in 1880, 549 in 1900, to more than 1,800 in 1920. For information on the increase in training programs, see Wendell W. Oderkirk, "Setting the Record Straight: A Recount of Late Nineteenth-Century Training Schools," *Journal of Nursing History* 1 (November 1985): 30–37; Council on Medical Education and Hospitals of the American Medical Association, "Third Presentation of Hospital Data," *Journal of the American Medical Association* 82 (1924): 118; May Ayres Burgess, *Nurses, Patients, and Pocketbooks: A Study of the Economics of Nursing* (New York: Committee on the Grading of Nursing Schools, 1928). For information on the increase in hospitals, see Joan E. Lynaugh, "From Respectable Domesticity to Medical Efficiency: The Changing Kansas City Hospital, 1875–1920," in *The American General Hospital: Communities and Social Contexts,* ed. Diana Elizabeth Long and Janet Golden (Ithaca, N.Y.: Cornell University Press, 1989), 21–39; Starr, *Transformation of Medicine,* chap. 4.

20. "Minutes of the Officers and Trustees," 1902, SL/UH Collection, MHS.

21. The exact figures include a mean time between application and admission of 110.9 days, reflecting an increase from 86.8 days (1897–1910) to 132.4 days (1924–1935). Unless otherwise stated, all figures cited in regard to the nurses of the St. Luke's Hospital Training School for Nurses are from the database described in chapter 1. SLHTS Collection, MHS.

22. See the discussion of this finding under the section "Rural Beginnings," later in this chapter.

23. John L. Frohnmayer, "The Captive Conscience: Teaching in an Age of Intellectual Intimidation," *National Teaching and Learning Forum* 7 (1998): 6. Frohnmayer is

the former chairman of the National Endowment for the Arts. In regard to contemporary teaching and evaluation, he adds, "We are afraid to speak frankly. We have forgotten that offense is inevitable and necessary if we are to express ourselves."

24. Such an assurance was asked of all applicants. See "Application Guidelines" and application forms, SLHTS Collection, MHS.

25. Edward J. Halloran, "Men in Nursing," in *Current Issues in Nursing*, ed. Joanne Comi McCloskey and Helen Kennedy Grace (Boston: Blackwell Scientific Publications, 1985), 969–78; Kalisch and Kalisch, *Advance of Nursing*, 627–35.

26. Judith Godden, "Victorian Influences on the Development of Nursing," in *Scholarship in the Discipline of Nursing*, ed. Genevieve Gray and Rosalie Pratt, 239–54 (New York: Churchill Livingstone, 1995); Judith Godden, "Nightingale's Legacy and Hours of Work," in *Nursing History and the Politics of Welfare*, ed. Anne Marie Rafferty, Jane Robinson, and Ruth Elkan (New York: Routledge, 1997), 184; Sandra Horton, "Feminine Authority and Social Order: Florence Nightingale's Conception of Nursing and Health Care," *Social Analysis* 15 (1984): 59–101.

27. Cited in Godden, "Victorian Influences."

28. Florence Nightingale, letter to Mary Jones (superintendent of St. John's nurses at University College Hospital, 1867), in *As Miss Nightingale Said . . .*, ed. Monica Baly (London: Scutari Press, 1991), 96.

29. Statistics are from the United States Public Use Samples, 1910 and 1940. In 1900, 5.3 percent of all nurses were men, including both "trained and untrained nurses" (1900 Public Use Sample). The 1910 United States Census actually differentiated between trained and "unspecified" nurses. Those in the latter category presumably received no formal training or, at most, only minimal formal training. The 1940 United States Census introduced the new category of practical nurse. As Philip and Beatrice Kalisch explain, these were mostly "self-styled" nurses with little or no formal training. Thus, both groups generally fit the term *untrained nurse*. In order to simplify terminology, *untrained nurse* is used in the text to refer to these groups. Also see Kalisch and Kalisch, *Advance of Nursing*, 2d ed., 558–60.

30. Mary Elizabeth Carnegie, *The Path We Tread: Blacks in Nursing, 1854–1984* (Philadelphia: J. B. Lippincott Company, 1986), 20–33. African American women were represented in nursing in the following percentages: in 1900, 8.5 percent of all nurses; in 1910, 1.0 percent of all trained nurses and 15.8 percent of "unspecified" and presumably untrained nurses; in 1950, 6.0 percent of trained nurses (source: United States Public Use Samples, 1900, 1910; figure for 1950 cited in Kalisch and Kalisch, 2d ed., *Advance of Nursing*, 608). Two other authors provide useful, related information: Vanessa Northington Gamble, *Making a Place for Ourselves: The Black Hospital Movement, 1920–1945* (New York: Oxford University Press, 1995); Susan L. Smith, *Sick and Tired of Being Sick and Tired: Black Women's Health Activism in America, 1890–1950* (Philadelphia: University of Pennsylvania Press, 1995). Gamble examines the movement to improve training and clinical facilities for black physicians and nurses and to improve care for blacks. Smith focuses on the relationship between black women's health activism and public health.

31. St. Luke's Hospital Patient Register, 1892–1937, SL/UH Collection, MHS.

32. "Minutes of the Ramsey County Graduate Nurses' Association," April 6, 1903 and May 1903, Minnesota Nurses' Association, Fourth District Collection, Minnesota

Historical Society, St. Paul, Minn., 62–64. Minnesota Nurses' Association, Fourth District Collection is hereafter cited as MNA/FD Collection.

33. Blanche M. Pinkus, "Rolling Along" (a history of the Ramsey County Graduate Nurses' Association), 1938, MNA/FD Collection.

34. "Minutes of the Ramsey County Graduate Nurses' Association," April 6, 1903 and May 1903, MNA/FD Collection, MHS, 62–64.

35. Ibid.

36. See for example Strachan, *Labour of Love*. Strachan focuses on nurses in Australia, although her observations apply generally. She writes, "Women were not perceived as breadwinners, with paid work existing only until marriage" (109). Louise C. Selanders also takes note of this in "Florence Nightingale: The Evolution and Social Impact of Feminist Values in Nursing," *Journal of Holistic Nursing* 16 (June 1998): 247–63. She notes that Nightingale viewed marriage as "the ultimate temporal prison for women" (256).

37. The exact percentages were widowed, 1.3 percent, and divorced or separated, 1.4 percent.

38. Application letters, January 13, 1931, n.d., January 27, 1931, file "M. Cartwright," Box 4, SLHTS Collection, MHS.

39. Letter from superintendent, January 1931, file "M. Cartwright," Box 4, SLHTS Collection, MHS.

40. Application letters, February 6, 1906, February 15, 1906, n.d., file "E. Claggett," Box 1, SLHTS Collection, MHS. See chapters 5 and 6 for further discussion of issues related to family and marriage.

41. Superintendent's notes, February 1906, file "E. Claggett," Box 1, SLHTS Collection, MHS.

42. Claudia Goldin, *Understanding the Gender Gap: An Economic History of American Women* (New York: Oxford University Press, 1990), 160–66.

43. Darlene Clark Hine, *Black Women in White: Racial Conflict and Cooperation in the Nursing Profession, 1890–1950* (Bloomington: Indiana University Press, 1989). See also Carnegie, *Path We Tread*.

44. This possibility is highlighted in Christine Bose, Roslyn Feldberg, and Natalie Sokoloff with the Women and Work Research Group, eds., *Hidden Aspects of Women's Work* (New York: Praeger, 1987).

45. "Annual Report of St. Luke's Hospital," 1892, SL/UH Collection, MHS; *Tenth Anniversary of The Swedish Hospital, 1898–1908* (Minneapolis: Swedish Hospital [on permanent deposit with MHS], 1908), 25.

46. "Announcement," brochures describing the training program, 1920, 1930, SL/UH Collection, MHS.

47. Isabel Maitland Stewart, *The Education of Nurses: Historical Foundations and Modern Trends* (New York: Macmillan, 1944), 153–54. Also see King, "Conflicting Interests," 131; Susan M. Reverby, *Ordered to Care: The Dilemma of American Nursing, 1850–1945* (Cambridge: Cambridge University Press, 1987), 85; Wendell W. Oderkirk, "'Organize or Perish': The Transformation of Nebraska Nursing Education, 1888–1941" (Ph.D. diss., University of Nebraska, 1988), 164.

48. "Annual Report(s) of St. Luke's Hospital," 1893, 1920, SL/UH Collection, MHS.

49. For example, as a member of the Undergraduate Admission and Progression

Committee at the University of Hawaii School of Nursing, colleagues and I reviewed fifty-three applications for twenty-five positions in the spring semester 1998 nursing class.

50. United States Census Office, *Eleventh Census of the U.S.: 1890* (Washington, D.C.: Government Printing Office, 1895c, 1897); United States Bureau of the Census, *Fourteenth Census of the U.S.: 1920* (Washington, D.C.: Government Printing Office, 1923).

51. See, for example, Reverby, *Ordered to Care,* 85.

52. Application letter, March 13, 1901, file "A. Lucken," Box 1, SLHTS Collection, MHS. Also see application letter, November 7, 1900, file "M. Johnson," Box 1, SLHTS Collection, MHS.

53. Application letter, August 11, 1913, file "A. Strand," SLHTS Collection, MHS.

54. Reference letter, August 8, 1913, file "A. Strand," Box 2, SLHTS Collection, MHS.

55. Reference letter, October 31, 1910, file "V. Spofford," Box 1, SLHTS Collection, MHS.

56. Reference letter, August 24, 1916, file "R. Lyon," Box 2, SLHTS Collection, MHS.

57. Application interview notes, August 1904, file "C. Mehnert," Box 1, SLHTS Collection, MHS.

58. Application letter, January 20, 1917, file "F. Kellar," Box 2, SLHTS Collection, MHS. Both this and the preceding record also show that admission of prospective nurses required the approval of both the hospital superintendent and the nursing superintendent.

59. Application letters, December 12, 1900 and May 26, 1901, file "M. Crowl," Box 1, SLHTS Collection, MHS.

60. Application letter, December 5, 1905, file "I. Schnepel," Box 5, SLHTS Collection, MHS.

61. Application letter, December 30, 1907, file "S. Rightmire," Box 5, SLHTS Collection, MHS.

62. Application letter, February 19, 1909, file "L. Reynolds," Box 5; application letter, April 10, 1912, file "R. Richardson," and Box 5; application letter, June 27, 1916, file "R. Johnson," Box 2, SLHTS Collection, MHS.

63. Application letter, 1917, file "G. Rothschild," Box 2, SLHTS Collection, MHS.

64. Superintendent's notes, 1917, file "G. Rothschild," Box 2, SLHTS Collection, MHS.

65. Reference letter, February 9, 1904, file "E. Burden," Box 1, SLHTS Collection, MHS.

66. Reference letter, October 25, 1899, file "F. Crosby," Box 1, SLHTS Collection, MHS.

67. Reference letter, October 10, 1907, file "R. Funk," Box 1, SLHTS Collection, MHS.

68. Reference letter, February 5, 1906, file "G. Funk," Box 1, SLHTS Collection, MHS. For another example see reference letter, August 10, 1905, file "M. Ensign," Box 1, SLHTS Collection, MHS.

69. Reference letter, 1921, file "A. Solberg," Box 5, SLHTS Collection, MHS.

70. Reference letter, February 27, 1932, file "M. Bruget, Box 4, SLHTS Collection, MHS.

71. Reference letter, n.d., file "M. Strand," Box 4, SLHTS Collection, MHS.

72. Ann Game and Rosemary Pringle. *Gender at Work* (Boston: George Allen and Unwin, 1983), 28.

73. Susan Lehrer, "A Living Wage Is for Men Only: Minimum Wage Legislation for Women, 1910–1925," in *Hidden Aspects of Women's Work,* ed. Christine Bose et al. (New York: Praeger, 1987), 206, citing C. W. Fulton, Brief for plaintiff in error, Records and Briefs of the Supreme Court, *Stettler* v. *O'Hara,* October term 1916–1917, Docket no. 25, no. 26, U.S. Supreme Court, 52.

74. Game and Pringle, *Gender at Work,* 28–30.

75. Ronnie J. Steinberg, "Gendered Instructions: Cultural Lag and Gender Bias in the Hay System of Job Evaluation," *Work and Occupations* 19 (November 1992): 387.

76. Cited in Strachan, *Labour of Love,* 10.

77. Cited in Bertha Estelle Merrill, *The Trek from Yesterday: A History of Organized Nursing in Minneapolis, 1883–1936* (Minneapolis: By the author [on permanent deposit with MHS], 1944), 57.

78. Karen Anne Wolf, ed., *Jo Ann Ashley: Selected Readings* (New York: NLN Press, 1997), 227, 231.

79. One variation to this approach is considering nursing as a domestic craft, a direct extension of women's activities in the home. Such an approach could conceivably lead to concealing or even dismissing the physical requirements of such a craft because they did not conform to a "real," translate to "masculine," craft. See Glenda Riley, "In or Out of the Historical Kitchen," *Minnesota History* 52 (summer 1990): 61–71. Riley carefully describes the nineteenth-century Midwestern tradition in which "women worked as domestic artisans in their homes, which also served as their workplaces or factories." She explains, "Rural women's writings overflow with details about whitewashing cabin walls, making medicines and treating the ill, making candles and soap, processing foods, cooking in open fireplaces or on small stoves, making cloth and clothing, and washing clothes" (63). An interesting speculation suggested by Riley's work is that, as time went on, rural women may have been more likely than urban women to maintain a view of nursing that was closer to the idea of hospital-based training, by virtue of their domestic artisan tradition.

80. For more specific figures see Thomas C. Olson, "The Women of St. Luke's and the Evolution of Nursing, 1892–1937" (Ph.D. diss., University of Minnesota, 1991), tables 22–23.

81. Examples of well-known studies that focus on the Northeast include Reverby, *Ordered to Care;* Mottus, *New York Nightingales;* and Nancy Tomes, "'Little World of Our Own': The Pennsylvania Hospital Training School for Nurses, 1895–1907," in *Women and Health in America: Historical Readings,* ed. Judith Walzer Leavitt (Madison: University of Wisconsin Press, 1984), 467–81.

82. Thomas J. Baerwald, "Forces at Work on the Landscape," in *Minnesota in a Century of Change: The State and Its People Since 1900,* ed. Clifford E. Clark Jr. (St. Paul: Minnesota Historical Society, 1989), 40.

83. Edward Eggleston, *The Mystery of Metropolisville* (New York: Orange Judd and Co., 1873).

84. Laura Ingalls Wilder, *On the Banks of Plum Creek* (New York: Harper and Row, 1953); idem, *By the Shores of Silver Lake* (New York: Harper and Row, 1953).

85. Sinclair Lewis, *Main Street* (New York: Harcourt, Brace and Howe, 1920); Garrison Keillor, *Lake Wobegon Days* (New York: Penguin, 1995).

86. This total is based on size of birthplace information from 505 St. Luke's nurses. Consistent with census definitions of the period, urban was viewed as a population of 2,500 or more; medium, 2,501 to 9,999; and rural, 2,500 or under. For source, see table 1. For more detailed information see Thomas Olson, *Women of St. Luke's,* table 2.

87. Reverby, *Ordered to Care,* 80–81. The same population distribution as described in the preceding note was used in Reverby's work.

88. This conclusion is based on information regarding size of address just prior to the start of training from 828 St. Luke's nurses. For source, see table 1. For more detailed information see Thomas Olson, *Women of St. Luke's,* table 3. In contrast to the conclusion here, Reverby found only a small increase in the percentage of women residing in rural areas at the time of admission to Boston Training Schools. Ibid., 210.

89. "Crops Excellent, Reports Indicate," *St. Paul Pioneer Press,* July 7, 1918, 2.

90. "Corn Reflects Drop in Feeding Operations," *St. Paul Pioneer Press,* February 1, 1931, 13.

91. Reverby, *Ordered to Care,* 81.

92. Correspondence, 1900, file "V. Book," Box 1, SLHTS Collection, MHS. 1900.

93. Blegen, *Minnesota: A History,* 295. For a more extensive discussion of transportation changes see John R. Borchert, "The Network of Urban Centers," in *Minnesota in a Century of Change: The State and Its People Since 1900,* ed. Clifford E. Clark Jr. (St. Paul: Minnesota Historical Society, 1989), 55–97.

94. William Watts Folwell, *A History of Minnesota,* vol. 3 (St. Paul: Minnesota Historical Society, 1969), 309.

95. John Borchert, "Urban Centers," 71; Chauncy D. Harris, "Agricultural Production in the United States: The Last Fifty Years and the Next," *Geographical Review* 60 (1970): 50–51.

96. Walsh, Eileen, "The Last Resort: Northern Minnesota Tourism and the Integration of Rural and Urban Worlds, 1900–1950" (Ph.D. diss., University of Minnesota, 1994). See chapter 5, "Tourism's Opportunities and Costs: Local Laborers."

97. Blegen, *Minnesota: A History,* 481; "Report Covering System and Operations," 1931, Department of Rural Credit Records, MHS.

98. Lucretia Delaney Himes, interview by author, tape recording, St. Paul, Minn., December 10, 1989.

99. For background on the resistance to paying nurses in training, see Helen E. Marshall, *Mary Adelaide Nutting: Pioneer of Modern Nursing* (Baltimore, Md.: Johns Hopkins University Press, 1972), 70–72; and Stewart, *Education of Nurses,* 160–64.

100. "Annual Report of St. Luke's Hospital," 1892, SL/UH Collection, MHS; "Annual Report(s) of Training Schools for Nurses," training program data reported to the New York Board of Nurse Examiners, 1909–1935, Box 1, SLHTS Collection, MHS.

101. Reference letter, June 27, 1916, file "L. Jones," Box 2, SLHTS Collection, MHS.

102. Report on St. Luke's Hospital Training School for Nurses, 1920, Box 19, Nurses Examiners Board, MHS.

103. Reference letters, August 17, 1918, August 21, 1918, and August 26, 1918, file "M. Hansen," Box 4, SLHTS Collection, MHS.

104. These totals are based on previous education information from 744 St. Luke's

nurses. For source, see table 1. For more detailed information see Thomas Olson, *Women of St. Luke's,* tables 4–5.

105. "Announcement," brochure describing the training program, 1924, SL/UH Collection, MHS.

106. United States Public Use Sample, 1940. For comparison, a comparable age range (18–30 years old) was used; the sample included 10.9 percent who had attended some college.

107. Committee for the Study of Nursing Education, Josephine Goldmark, secretary, *Nursing and Nursing Education in the United States* (New York: Macmillan, 1923). An argument similar to the one here would also apply to the absence of any apparent relationship between changes at St. Luke's and other reform efforts sponsored by nursing leaders, such as the Committee on Education, *Standard Curriculum for Schools of Nursing* (New York: National League for Nursing Education, 1917). It should be noted that St. Luke's was accredited by the New York Board of Nurse Examiners and the Minnesota Board of Nurse Examiners (Box 1, SLHTS Collection, MHS; and Minnesota Board of Nurse Examiners Collection, MHS; see chapter 4 for a more thorough discussion of accreditation).

108. Cynthia A. Connolly, "Hampton, Nutting, and Rival Gospels at The Johns Hopkins Hospital and Training School for Nurses, 1889–1906," *Image: Journal of Nursing Scholarship* 30 (first quarter 1998): 24. Also see Reverby, *Ordered to Care,* chap. 4.

109. Stewart, *Education of Nurses,* 153.

110. Charles E. Rosenberg, *The Care of Strangers* (Cambridge, England: Cambridge University Press, 1987); Connolly, "Hampton, Nutting, and Rival Gospels," 24.

111. Reference letters, November 2, 1900 and November 7, 1900, file "M. Johnson," Box 1, SLHTS Collection, MHS.

112. Application letter and superintendent's notes, September 14, 1903, file "M. Dyer," Box 1, SLHTS Collection, MHS.

113. Reference letter, June 1912, file "C. Hanson," Box 2, SLHTS Collection, MHS.

114. Reference letter, September 2, 1913, file "M. Brooks," Box 2; reference letter, March 10, 1900, file "C. Paden," Box 1; reference letter, June 1927, file "L. Hansen," Box 4; reference letter, June 7, 1912, file "C. Hanson," Box 1; reference letter, August 8, 1914, file "D. Cashman," Box 2; and reference letter, January 3, 1922, file "E. Swanson," Box 5, SLHTS Collection, MHS. The emphasis on common sense and practicality is also reinforced by the way in which job experience was used to make up for somehow falling short of educational expectations. For instance, the lack of formal education for an applicant in 1899 was allayed by the fact that she "has been practicing as (a) professional nurse in and around Valley City for some time . . ." (reference letter, November 25, 1900, file "A. Liverson," Box 1, SLHTS Collection, MHS). An applicant wrote in 1903, "I wish I might say my education was more efficient than it is." This deficiency, however, was more than made up by experience assisting two physicians, as well as "having been housekeeper for my brothers and sisters for the past eight years" (application letter, September 10, 1903, file "M. McKay," Box 1, SLHTS Collection, MHS). Also see application letter, January 13, 1931, file "M. Cartwright," Box 4, SLHTS Collection, MHS.

115. "Editorially Speaking," *Trained Nurse and Hospital Review* 31 (August 1903): 103–4. For a similar example see Florence M. Joslin, "The Ideal Nurse," *Trained Nurse and Hospital Review* 52 (January 1914): 44.

116. Shirley C. Titus and Margaret Huey, "Appointment to the Faculty," *American Journal of Nursing* 36 (June 1936): 597–601.

117. Connolly, "Hampton, Nutting, and Rival Gospels," 23–29.

118. Stewart, *The Education of Nurses,* 153.

119. This total is based on previous training information from 744 St. Luke's nurses. Overall, 22.9 percent of those entering St. Luke's during 1897–1910 reported previous training experience, compared to 29.3 percent of those entering during 1911–1923 and 13.1 percent of those entering during 1924–1935. Normal school accounted for 40.9 percent of the previous training, followed by clerical school (19.9 percent), prior nurses' training elsewhere (20.5 percent), and other types of training (18.7 percent). For source, see table 1. For more detailed information see Thomas Olson, *Women of St. Luke's,* table 5.

120. Clarke A. Chambers, "Educating for the Future," in *Minnesota in a Century of Change: The State and Its People Since 1900,* ed. Clifford E. Clark Jr. (St. Paul: Minnesota Historical Society Press, 1989), 476.

121. The reduction of training programs not only in Minnesota, but nationwide, began in 1929 and continued for the next ten years. Many of the sponsoring hospitals also closed their doors as the result of financial problems. For more detailed information see Stewart, *Education of Nurses,* 248–50.

122. Various interview and application notes, Boxes 4, SLHTS Collection, MHS.

123. Kunz, *Saint Paul,* 71.

124. Ibid.

125. Ibid.

126. Ibid.

127. Ibid, 71–72. For additional information related to this citation see Henry Castle, *History of St. Paul and Vicinity: A Chronicle of Progress and Narrative Account of the Industries, Institutions and People of the City and Its Tributary Territory* (New York: Lewis Publishing Company, 1912).

128. This total is based on previous occupation information from 684 St. Luke's nurses. For source, see table 1. For more detailed information see Thomas Olson, *Women of St. Luke's,* table 6.

129. For more specific data regarding the nurses' previous occupations see Thomas Olson, *Women of St. Luke's,* table 6. Among the additional findings, more than one in ten of the women (13 percent) had two or more jobs prior to coming to St. Luke's.

130. For a detailed explanation of the occupational classification used here see Tom Olson, "The Women of St. Luke's and the Occupational Evolution of Nursing, 1897–1915," *Mid-America: An Historical Review* 73 (April–July 1991): 135–50. Categories and occupations were validated by an independent reviewer. Also refer to Margo Conk Anderson, "Occupational Classification in the United States Census: 1870–1940," *Journal of Interdisciplinary History* 9, no. 1 (1978): 111–30; Virginia Jelatis, "The Measurement of Changing Occupational Structure in Public Use Samples, 1880–1980," paper presented at the Fifteenth Annual Meeting of the Social Science History Association, Minneapolis, Minn., October 18–21, 1990.

131. Ruth Houlton, *The Profession of Nursing* (Minneapolis: Woman's Occupational Bureau, 1930), 10.

132. Kirk Jeffrey, "The Major Manufacturers: From Food and Forest Products to High Technology," in *Minnesota in a Century of Change: The State and Its People Since 1900,* ed. Clifford E. Clark Jr. (St. Paul: Minnesota Historical Society Press, 1989), 224.

133. Marjorie Bingham, "Keeping at It: Minnesota Women," in *Minnesota in a Century of Change: The State and Its People Since 1900,* ed. Clifford E. Clark Jr. (St. Paul: Minnesota Historical Society Press, 1989), 435.

134. Minnesota Bureau of Labor, Commerce and Industry, Woman's Department, *First Biennial Report, 1907–1908* (St. Paul: Willwerscheid and Roith, 1909), 14.

135. [Mrs. Perry Starkweather], "Department of Women and Children," in Minnesota Bureau of Labor, Industries and Commerce, *Twelfth Biennial Report, 1909–1910* (St. Paul: Willwerscheid and Roith, 1910), 607.

136. Resolution cited in Fletcher Harper Swift, "The Increasing Professionalization of Educational Workers," in *Changing Educational World,* ed. Alvin C. Eurich (Minneapolis: University of Minnesota Press, 1931), 205.

137. Chambers, "Educating for the Future," 480–82; Jean H. Alexander, "Chronological Outline of the Development of Public Education in Minnesota," in *Changing Educational World,* ed. Alvin C. Eurich (Minneapolis: University of Minnesota Press, 1931), 249–57.

138. The inclusion of nurses in this category assumes their possession of specific skills, in contrast to placing them in the laborers category.

139. Women were not required to complete nurse's training in order to practice nursing. Registration and licensure for nurses did not become mandatory in Minnesota until 1960.

140. Burgess, *Nurses and Pocketbooks,* 197–202, 340; Barbara Melosh, *"The Physician's Hand": Work Culture and Conflict in American Nursing* (Philadelphia: Temple University Press, 1982), 77–79.

141. Merrill, *The Trek from Yesterday,* 14.

142. Monica Baly, ed., *As Miss Nightingale Said . . .* (London: Scutari Press, 1991), 63.

143. Robert Smuts, *Women and Work in America* (New York: Columbia University Press, 1959), 80–81. Smuts also suggests that the strains in rural teaching were different than those in nursing. For additional discussion of women and teaching see Michael Apple, "Teaching and 'Women's Work,'" *Teachers College Record* 86 (1985): 455–73; and Jean Christie, "Sarah Christie Steven, Schoolwoman," *Minnesota History* 48 (summer 1983): 245–62.

144. Application letter, May 6, 1918, file "N. Swenson," Box 5, SLHTS, MHS.

145. Angel Kwolek-Folland, "Gender, Self, and Work in the Life Insurance Industry, 1880–1930," in *Work Engendered: Toward a New History of American Labor,* ed. Ava Baron (Ithaca, N.Y.: Cornell University Press, 1991), 179.

146. Goldin, *Gender Gap,* 3–9, 75–77. Also see Kessler-Harris, Alice, *Women Have Always Worked: A Historical Overview* (New York: The Feminist Press, 1981); Ileen A. DeVault, "'Give the Boys a Trade': Gender and Job Choice in the 1890s," in Baron, *Work Engendered,* 191–215.

147. Houlton, *Profession of Nursing,* 3.

Notes to Chapter 3

1. Application letter, December 15, 1911, file "A. Wilson," Box 1, St. Luke's Hospital Training School Collection, Minnesota Historical Society, St. Paul, Minn. This collection is hereafter cited as SLHTS Collection, MHS.

2. Application letter and application form, May 16, 1929, file "L. Sommerfeld," Box 3, SLHTS Collection, MHS.

3. "Big Buyers Ready to Enter Market, Gotham Bankers Say After Second Crash," *St. Paul Pioneer Press,* October 7, 1929, 1.

4. "Northwest Conditions Termed Satisfactory," *St. Paul Pioneer Press,* October 6, 1929, 1.

5. "Annual Report(s) of St. Luke's Hospital," 1893, 1920, St. Luke's/United Hospital Collection, Minnesota Historical Society, St. Paul, Minn. This collection is hereafter cited as SL/UH Collection, MHS. Refer also to chapter 2.

6. Beverly Boutilier, "Helpers or Heroines? The National Council of Women, Nursing, and 'Woman's Work' in Late Victorian Canada," in *Caring and Curing: Historical Perspectives on Women and Healing in Canada,* ed. Dianne Dodd and Deborah Gorham (Ottawa: University of Ottawa Press, 1994), 29. Boutilier adds that "an ideal of 'feminine' self-sacrifice and self-forgetfulness still undergirded . . . the construction of nursing as one of the 'female' professions" (ibid., 41).

7. Stella Bingham, *Ministering Angels* (London: Osprey Publishing, 1979); Esther Ring Mulvany, *Lamps Still Aglow: A History of Kansas Nursing* (North Newton, Kans.: Mennonite Press, 1976). Refer also to any of the early accounts of nursing for a general description of the standard view of the religious and military antecedents of organized nursing. See, for example, Lavinia L. Dock and Isabel Maitland Stewart, *A Short History of Nursing* (New York: G. P. Putnam's Sons, 1920), chaps. 3–4.

8. Philip A. Kalisch and Beatrice J. Kalisch, "Slaves, Servants, or Saints? An Analysis of the System of Nurse Training in the United States, 1873–1948," *Nursing Forum* 14 (1975): 223–63. See also Siobhan Nelson, *Say Little, Do Much: Nurses, Nuns, and Hospitals in the Nineteenth Century* (Philadelphia: University of Pennsylvania Press, 2001). Nelson argues that religious nursing was "formative of professional nursing in profound and far-reaching ways" (p. 1).

9. Ibid. This account is also typical in suggesting that training programs were extensions of early religious movements which, admittedly, incorporated elements of harsh, military-style discipline.

10. Cynthia Q. Woods, "From Individual Dedication to Social Activism: Historical Development of Nursing Professionalism," in *Nursing History: The State of the Art,* ed. Christopher Maggs (Wolfeboro, N.H.: Croom Helm, 1987), 153–55. Woods also explains that the nursing's saintly ideal underlies its reliance on "common sense individualism," which further frustrated professional development.

11. Nancy Johnston Hall and Mary Bround Smith, *Traditions United: The History of St. Luke's and Charles T. Miller Hospitals and Their Service to St. Paul* (St. Paul: United Hospital Foundation, , 1987), 5. Note that Van Ingen took his text from 1 Cor. 13:1.

12. June Drenning Holmquist, *They Chose Minnesota: A Survey of the State's Ethnic Groups* (St. Paul: Minnesota Historical Society Press, 1981).

13. Virginia Brainard Kunz, *Saint Paul: The First 150 Years* (St. Paul: Saint Paul Foundation, 1991), 48.

14. William C. Pope, *The Church in St. Paul* (St. Paul: Minnesota Historical Society, 1911); Rev. George C. Tanner, *Fifty Years of Church Work in the Diocese of Minnesota, 1857–1907* (St. Paul: The Committee, 1909); Hall and Smith, *Traditions United;* "A History of St. Luke's," apparently written by a member of the alumnae association, [ca. 1940], SL/UH Collection, MHS. Note that St. Luke's Hospital actually opened in 1857 as the Christ Church Orphan's Home and Hospital, later renamed the Church Hospital and Orphan's Home of St. Paul, and renamed again in 1877 as the St. Luke's Hospital. Average cost per week of patients in 1877 was $5.64.

15. Joan E. Lynaugh, "From Respectable Domesticity to Medical Efficiency: The Changing Kansas City Hospital, 1875–1920," in *The American General Hospital: Communities and Social Contexts,* ed. Diana Elizabeth Long and Janet Golden (Ithaca, N.Y.: Cornell University Press, 1989), 27.

16. Judith Godden, "Victorian Influences on the Development of Nursing," in *Scholarship in the Discipline of Nursing,* ed. Genevieve Gray and Rosalie Pratt, 239–54 (New York: Churchill Livingstone, 1995), 251.

17. Nurses' files, STLHS Collection, MHS. For a complete breakdown of religious affiliation by time period see Thomas Olson, *Women of St. Luke's,* table 8.

18. These totals are based on religious background information from 753 St. Luke's nurses. For source, see table 1. For more detailed information see Thomas Olson, *Women of St. Luke's,* table 8.

19. Ibid.

20. Henry Castle, *History of St. Paul and Vicinity: A Chronicle of Progress and Narrative Account of the Industries, Institutions and People of the City and Its Tributary Territory* (New York: Lewis Publishing Company, 1912); Kunz, *Saint Paul.* For a broader discussion of religion in Minnesota see Theodore Blegen, *Minnesota: A History of the State* (Minneapolis: University of Minnesota Press, 1975), 206–7, 307; and Richard M. Chapman, "Religious Belief and Behavior," in *Minnesota in a Century of Change: The State and Its People Since 1900,* ed. Clifford E. Clark Jr. (St. Paul: Minnesota Historical Society Press, 1990), 507–38.

21. Nurses' files, STLHS Collection, MHS.

22. For a complete breakdown of motivating factors for choosing St. Luke's see Thomas Olson, *Women of St. Luke's,* table 29. It is noteworthy that the applicants' statements regarding their motivation to become trained nurses, and specifically to enter St. Luke's, suggest that they had considerable awareness regarding the nature of nursing work and training.

23. For a complete breakdown of motivating factors for entering nurses' training see Thomas Olson, *Women of St. Luke's,* table 28.

24. Note that the percentage of those who denied or did not mention religion in the application process actually decreased after 1910, which like the findings in regard to age and education suggests a tightening rather than loosening of entrance standards. Still, "nonprofessed" individuals maintained a sizable presence throughout the school's existence (see Thomas Olson, *Women of St. Luke's,* table 8).

25. "Minutes of the Board of Trustees and Managers," 1902–1912, SL/UH Collection, MHS, 14–17.

26. Ibid.

27. Ibid.

28. Dorothy Slocum, interview by Nancy Johnston Hall, 1987, Transcript, SL/UH Collection, MHS.

29. "Annual Report of St. Luke's Hospital," 1920, SL/UH Collection, MHS.

30. Reference letter, November 16, 1899, file "M. McEwan," Box, SLHTS Collection, MHS.

31. Reference letters, December 7, 1900 and December 13, 1900, file "M. Campeau," Box 1; reference letter, ca. 1909, file "J. Templeman," Box 1; reference letter, March 27, 1918, file "M. Baer," Box 2; reference letter, July 26, 1927, file "A. Dahl," Box 3; and reference letter, March 16, 1932, file "E. Schutt," Box 5, SLHTS Collection, MHS.

32. Wendell W. Oderkirk, "'Organize or Perish': The Transformation of Nebraska Nursing Education, 1888–1941" (Ph.D. diss., University of Nebraska, 1988), 214–17.

33. Susan M. Reverby, *Ordered to Care: The Dilemma of American Nursing, 1850–1945* (Cambridge: Cambridge University Press, 1987), 47. Reverby's contention that character was the essential skill of nursing will be addressed further, particularly in discussing the work of nursing in chapter 4.

34. Ibid., 50.

35. "St. Paul Women Rally to Call for Great Increase in Knitting," and "Protection of Girls Planned in Capital," *St. Paul Pioneer Press,* July 7, 1918, 4, 10.

36. Arthur W. Calhoun, *A Social History of the American Family* (Cleveland, 1919), 3:111.

37. Minnesota Bureau of Labor, *Ninth Biennial Report,* 1903–1904, 1:129, cited in Lynn Weiner, "Our Sister's Keepers: The Minneapolis Women's Christian Association and Housing for Working Women," *Minnesota History* 46, no. 5 (spring 1979): 189–200. Also see Smuts, Robert, *Women and Work in America* (New York: Columbia University Press, 1959), 118, chap. passim; and Harriet Bradley, *Men's Work, Women's Work: A Sociological History of the Sexual Division of Labour in Employment* (Cambridge, UK: Polity Press, 1989), 216–17; Regina Markell Morantz-Sanchez, *Sympathy and Science: Women Physicians in American Medicine* (New York: Oxford University Press, 1985), 106, 226–28, 289; Amy Gilman, "'Cogs to the Wheels': The Ideology of Women's Work in Mid-19th-Century Fiction," in *Hidden Aspects of Women's Work,* ed. Christine Bose et al. (New York: Praeger Publishers, 1987), 116–34, and Susan Lehrer, "A Living Wage Is for Men Only: Minimum Wage Legislation for Women, 1910–1925," in *Hidden Aspects of Women's Work,* ed. Bose et al.

38. Minnesota Bureau of Labor, *Ninth Biennial Report,* 1903–1904.

39. "Wage Purity War on Wickedness," *St. Paul Pioneer Press,* October 1, 1910, 12.

40. Arthur J. Larsen, ed., *Crusader and Feminist: Letters of Jane Grey Swisshelm, 1858–1865* (St. Paul: Minnesota Historical Society, 1934), 311.

41. Reference letter, November 19, 1910, file "V. Spofford," Box 5, SLHTS Collection, MHS.

42. Reference letter, March 13, 1915, file "J. Wilson," Box 2, SLHTS Collection, MHS.

43. Reference letter, July 6, 1927, file "M. Campbell," Box 4, SLHTS Collection, MHS.

44. Reference letter, April 11, 1928, file "L. Hansen," Box 4, SLHTS Collection, MHS.

45. "To Bob or Not to Bob," *St. Paul Pioneer Press,* October 1, 1924, 1.

46. Reference letter, February 12, 1932, file "M. Schell," Box 4, SLHTS Collection, MHS. In measuring the overall importance of the question about bobbed hair, one

must consider that women were admitted to the training program even if they answered yes to this question. It should also be noted that fewer references emphasized moral character as time went on, though what was emphasized remained the same. Further, exceptions were made to general moral expectations (e.g., acceptance of divorced women, as well as one individual who was open about receiving treatment for lues, i.e., syphilis).

47. The possibility that some of the actual experiences of nursing have been masked by the rhetoric of saintly nursing is more fully addressed in chapter 4.

48. Personality is defined according to Webster's shared meaning element: "the dominant qualities that distinguish a person" (*Webster's New Collegiate Dictionary,* 1976).

49. Application letter, December 15, 1911, file "A. Wilson," Box 1, SLHTS Collection, MHS.

50. Application letter, May 4, 1912, file "E. Carroll," Box 1, SLHTS Collection, MHS.

51. Reference letter, February 21, 1906, file "I. Solberg," Box 1, SLHTS Collection, MHS.

52. Reference letter, February 19, 1900, file "M. Farrington," Box 1, SLHTS Collection, MHS.

53. Application letter, December 26, 1909, file "E. Beatty," Box 4, SLHTS Collection, MHS.

54. Application letter, 1917, file "G. Anderson," Box 2, SLHTS Collection, MHS. Also see reference letter, June 27, 1916, file "E. Jones"; Box 2; and reference letter, May 15, 1931, file "H. Hone," Box 4, SLHTS Collection, MHS.

55. Reference letter, February 23, 1906, file "G. Funk," Box 1; reference letter, September 7, 1913, file "P. Anderson," Box 2; reference letter, March 13, 1915, file "J. Wilson," Box 2; reference letter, June 30, 1916, file "R. Johnson," Box 2; reference letter, May 5, 1930, file "F. Quimby," Box 5; reference letter, June 4, 1931, file "P. Mommsen," Box 5; and reference letter, n.d., file "A. Yde," Box 5, SLHTS Collection, MHS.

56. Application letter, 1917, file "H. Bennett," Box 4, SLHTS Collection, MHS.

57. Reference letter, February 26, 1933, file "E. Newman," Box 4, SLHTS Collection, MHS.

58. Kalisch and Kalisch, "Slaves or Saints," 225; Ashley, Jo Ann, *Hospitals, Paternalism and the Role of the Nurse* (New York: Teachers College Press, 1976),18; Susan Reverby, "The Search for the Hospital Yardstick: Nursing and the Rationalization of Hospital Work," in *Sickness and Health in America: Readings in the History of Medicine and Public Health,* 2d ed., ed. Judith Walzer Leavitt and Ronald L. Numbers (Madison: University of Wisconsin Press, 1985), 208.

59. St. Luke's Hospital Training School for Nurses folder, MBNE Collection, MHS. Refer also to the related discussion and notes in the preface.

60. See chapter 7 for a more complete discussion of this topic.

61. Quoted phrase is from a description of St. Luke's nurses in the St. Luke's Training School for Nurses folder, MBNE Collection, MHS.

62. Elizabeth Arsenault, "As I See It," *American Nurse* 24, no. 10 (November–December 1992): 4, 10.

63. Joan Wallach Scott, *Gender and the Politics of History* (New York: Columbia University Press, 1988), 63.

64. Barbara Melosh, *"The Physician's Hand": Work Culture and Conflict in American Nursing* (Philadelphia: Temple University Press, 1982), 48.

65. Reference letter, April 21 1910, file "G. Ueland," Box 5, SLHTS Collection, MHS.

66. Application letter, September 10, 1903, file "M. McKay," Box 1, SLHTS Collection, MHS.

67. Reference letter, October 31, 1910, file "V. Spofford," Box 5, SLHTS Collection, MHS.

68. Application letter, May 26, 1929, file "L. Sommerfeld," Box 3, SLHTS Collection, MHS.

69. Various trainee files, SLHTS Collection, MHS. Note that the phrase "practical skill(s)" was used in the files interchangeably with "nursing skill(s)" and the "skill(s) of nursing."

70. Application letter, February 23, 1900, file "E. Mallough," Box 1, SLHTS Collection, MHS.

71. Application letter, April 23, 1924, file "L. Jarvinen," Box 3, SLHTS Collection, MHS.

72. Application letter, June 14, 1910, file "E. Estabrook," Box 1, SLHTS Collection, MHS.

73. Reference letter, May 23, 1901, file "M. Price," Box 1, SLHTS Collection, MHS.

74. Application letter, July 20, 1902, file "L. Baker," Box 1, SLHTS Collection, MHS.

75. Reference letter, July 21, 1904, file "C. Mehnert," Box 1, SLHTS Collection, MHS.

76. Application letter, August 1909, file "E. Schoch," Box 5, SLHTS Collection, MHS. Although the probationary period varied somewhat at St. Luke's, it generally spanned six weeks, consistent with other training programs (see Philip A. Kalisch and Beatrice J. Kalisch, *The Advance of American Nursing,* 3d ed. [Philadelphia: J. B. Lippincott Company, 1995], 126–127).

77. Application letter, May 31, 1904, file "E. Man," Box 5, SLHTS Collection, MHS.

78. Application letter, August 27, 1912, file "M. Crary," Box 4, SLHTS Collection, MHS.

79. For example, in 1897 Miss Helen G. Hill changed her position as training superintendent to that of hospital superintendent, followed by similar switches by Margaret Crowl in 1916 and J. E. Catton in 1918. Occasionally, one individual would also occupy both positions, such as Grace Scott did in 1930.

80. Application form, February 12, 1924, file "J. Johnston," Box 4, SLHTS Collection, MHS.

81. Reference letter, n.d., file "C. Peterson," Box 4, SLHTS Collection, MHS. For an additional example see reference letter, June 22, 1907, file "B. Burrows," Box 2, SLHTS Collection, MHS.

82. DeVault, "Give the Boys a Trade," 206. While the apprenticeship of steamfitters and plumbers might have been more or less exacting than other trades, the emphasis on learning by practical experience remained a common thread.

83. Reference letter, February 27, 1902, file "D. Sweeney," Box 1, SLHTS Collection, MHS.

84. Reference letter, June 14, 1930, file "M. Turek," Box 5, SLHTS Collection, MHS.

85. Reference letter, September 3, 1902, file "B. Temple," Box 1, SLHTS Collection, MHS.

86. Application letter, January 3, 1912, file "A. Grasmoen," Box 4, SLHTS Collection, MHS.

87. Application letter, September 10, 1900, file "G. Westman," Box 1, SLHTS Collection, MHS.

88. Application letter, March 6, 1920, file "C. Ball," Box 3, SLHTS Collection MHS.

89. This payment amount is similar to that of other schools. See, for example, Pat Gaarder and Tracey Baker, *From Stripes to Whites: A History of the Swedish Hospital School of Nursing, 1899–1973* (Minneapolis: Alumnae Association, 1980), 13. Refer also to Thomas Olson, *Women of St. Luke's,* table 27.

90. David Montgomery, *The Fall of the House of Labor: The Workplace, the State, and American Labor Activism, 1865–1925* (New York: Cambridge University Press, 1987), 185.

91. Application letter, March 5, 1902, file "D. Sweeney," Box 1, SLHTS Collection, MHS.

92. Victor Cohn, *Sister Kenny: The Woman Who Challenged the Doctors* (Minneapolis: University of Minnesota Press), 1975; Peg Meier, "When Sister Kenny Came to Minneapolis," *Minneapolis Star Tribune* (December 17, 1992): sec. E, 1–3.

93. Celia Davies, *Gender and the Professional Predicament in Nursing* (Philadelphia: Open University Press, 1995), 24. Davies' ideas are based on a wide critique of feminist scholarship, including Carol Gilligan, *In a Different Voice* (Cambridge, Mass.: Harvard University Press, 1982); Nancy Chodorow, *Feminism and Psychoanalytic Theory* (London: Yale University Press, 1989); Sandra Harding, *The Science Question in Feminism* (Milton Keynes: Open University Press, 1986); Roslyn W. Bologh, *Love or Greatness: Max Weber and Masculine Thinking—A Feminist Inquiry* (London: Unwin Hyman, 1990); Luce Irigaray, *Je, Tu, Vous: Toward a Culture of Difference* (London: Routledge, 1993).

94. Davies, *Gender and the Professional,* 28–29.

95. Bologh, *Love or Greatness,* 15.

96. Ibid.

97. See, for example, Ashley, *Hospitals, Paternalism;* Reverby, *Ordered to Care;* Patricia M. Schwirian, *Professionalization of Nursing: Current Issues and Trends* (Philadelphia: Lippincott, 1998). Ashley's book is a particularly useful example of a work that narrowly concentrates on the oppression of early nurses within the general framework of professionalization.

98. Ashley, *Hospitals, Paternalism,* 76, 101. The thoroughness with which the medical elite was able to block the professionalizing strategies of their counterparts in nursing, the elite of a separate occupation, also testifies to the gender-based inequality that existed during this period. Unfortunately, accounts of nursing history seldom move beyond this fact in attempting to explain the occupational evolution of nursing.

99. Judith Moore, *A Zeal for Responsibility: The Struggle for Professional Nursing in Victorian England, 1868–1883* (Athens: University of Georgia Press, 1988), xi.

100. For background on this issue see Melosh, *"The Physician's Hand,"* 20; Kathleen Cannings and William Lazonick, "The Development of the Nursing Labor Force in the United States: A Basic Analysis," *International Journal of Health Services* 5 (1975): 185–216; Victoria T. Grando, "Class Status Among Student Nurses at the University of Kansas School of Nursing, 1907–1929," paper presented at the Eighth Annual Conference on Nursing History, San Francisco, September 28–30, 1991; Moore, *Zeal for Responsibility.*

101. Burgess, "Nurses, Patients," 300. Note that the Grading Committee project, in which Burgess participated, actually began in 1926.

102. Ibid., 300–1.

103. Ibid., 301.

104. Ibid.

105. Ibid.

106. It is important to note that most of the evidence for this two-tier system of nursing work and training in the United States relies on anecdotal evidence from elite training programs in the North East, rather than systematic evidence or evidence from other geographic areas. See Reverby, *Ordered to Care,* 87.

107. The exact percentage is 43.4 percent. See Tom Olson, "Women of St. Luke's and the Occupational," 146–48.

108. Sharon Sassler and Michael J. White, "Ethnicity, Gender, and Social Mobility in 1910," *Social Science History* 21 (fall 1997): 347.

109. These two areas, social positions and shared dispositions, represent separate levels in the formulation of class and serve to define this concept here. See also Mathew Sobek, "Class Analysis and the U.S. Census Public Use Samples," *Historical Methods* 24 (fall 1991): 171–82; Ira Katznelson, "Working-Class Formation: Constructing Cases and Comparisons," in *Working-Class Formation: Nineteenth-Century Patterns in Western Europe and the United States,* ed. Ira Katznelson and Aristide R. Zolberg (Princeton: Princeton University Press, 1986), 3–41.

110. For a detailed breakdown and description of the occupation classification used in this work see Tom Olson, "Women of St. Luke's and the Occupational," 139. Refer also to the related discussion in chapter 2.

111. United States Public Use Sample, 1910.

112. See the related discussion chapter 2 regarding the separation of trained and untrained nurses in the 1910 United States Census.

113. See also Tom Olson, "Women of St. Luke's and the Occupational"; and DeVault, "Give the Boys a Trade," 193.

114. Totals in this paragraph are based on occupational information from 1,230 references. For source, see table 1. For a detailed breakdown and description of the occupations of references see Tom Olson, "Women of St. Luke's and the Occupational," 149.

115. Burgess, "Nurses, Patients," 300.

116. Joan Wallach Scott, "Gender: A Useful Category of Historical Analysis," *American Historical Review* 91 (December 1986): 1053–75.

117. Patricia D'Antonio, "Revisiting and Rethinking the Rewriting of Nursing History," *Bulletin of the History of Medicine* 73 (1999): 280. See also Patricia D'Antonio, "Rethinking the Rewriting of Nursing History," *Chronicle* 9 (spring 1998): 4.

118. This last fact helps to explain the greater emphasis on exploitation in thinking about nursing from the standpoint of professionalization rather than a craft.

119. Barbara Melosh, "Apprenticeship Culture and Nurses' Resistance to Professionalization," in *Alternative Conceptions of Work and Society: Implications for Professional Nursing,* ed. Carol A. Lindeman (Washington, D.C.: American Association of Colleges of Nursing, 1988), 34–35. See also Margaret Bayldon, "Diploma Schools: The First Century," *RN* 36 (February 1973): 33–48.

NOTES TO CHAPTER 4

1. Grace Peter, nee Bakke, interviews by author, tape recording, Willmar, Minn., November 25, 1989 and April 1, 1990.

2. . This scenario is drawn from the file of "M. Young," Box 5, and other trainees, St. Luke's Hospital Training School Collection, Minnesota Historical Society, St. Paul, Minn. This collection is hereafter cited as SLHTS Collection, MHS. Note that the lack of religious emphasis is consistent with findings in chapter 3. Minimal religious observances included a five-minute chapel service held each day, with the exception of a half-hour service on Wednesdays.

3. "Italians Gain Advantage by Surprise Onslaught," *St. Paul Pioneer Press,* July 1, 1918, 1; "U.S. Airmen Victors in Fierce Half Hour Fight," *St. Paul Pioneer Press,* July 3, 1918, 1; "American Troops in France," *St. Paul Pioneer Press,* July 3, 1918, 1. The war-related need for nurses influenced the choice of at least some of the women to enter training. See, for example, application letter, November 3, 1918, file "M. Bear," Box 2, SLHTS Collection, MHS.

4. "Mothers Here Lack Patriotism," *St. Paul Pioneer Press,* July 10, 1918, 5.

5. "New Party Is Forming; May Invade State," *St. Paul Pioneer Press,* July 1, 1918, 1.

6. "Guard Closes Blooming Prairie Bars," *St. Paul Pioneer Press,* July 2, 1918, 1.

7. Application letter, February 17, 1918, file "M. Young," Box 5, SLHTS Collection, MHS.

8. All figures involving time spent on duty are drawn from the "monthly records," listings of the time in training and practical assignments of each trainee, Boxes 1–5, SLHTS Collection, MHS. Note that total time in the program was based on generally accepted norms for training, rather than state or nationally mandated totals. For additional discussion of this issue, as well as a more detailed listing of total time spent on duty, see Tom Olson, "Apprenticeship and Exploitation: An Analysis of the Work Pattern of Nurses in Training, 1897–1937," *Social Science History* 17 (winter 1993), 559–76.

9. Janet Wilson James, "Isabel Hampton and the Professionalization of Nursing," in *The Therapeutic Revolution: Essays in the Social History of American Medicine,* ed. M. J. Vogel and C. E. Rosenberg (Philadelphia: University of Pennsylvania Press, 1979), 224; Isabel Maitland Stewart, *The Education of Nurses: Historical Foundations and Modern Trends* (New York: Macmillan, 1944), 154–56; Isabel Hampton Robb, *Educational Standards for Nurses with Other Addresses on Nursing Subjects* (Cleveland: E. C. Koeckert, 1905/1907), 59. Note that Hampton became Hampton Robb after her marriage in 1894 to Dr. Hunter Robb.

10. Cynthia A. Connolly, "Hampton, Nutting, and Rival Gospels at The Johns Hopkins Hospital and Training School for Nurses, 1889–1906," *Image: Journal of Nursing Scholarship* 30 (first quarter 1998): 23–29; Isabel A. Hampton, "Educational Standards for Nurses," in *Nursing of the Sick (Papers presented at the International Congress of Charities, Correction, and Philanthropy) Held in Chicago, 1893* (New York: McGraw-Hill, 1893), 1–12.

11. Connolly, "Hampton, Nutting, and Rival Gospels"; Mary Adelaide Nutting, *A Sound Economic Basis for Schools of Nursing and Other Addresses* (New York: G.P. Putnam's, 1926), 339–50.

12. "Minutes of the Officers and Visitors," 1897–1902, St. Luke's/United Hospital

Collection, Minnesota Historical Society, St. Paul, Minn, 32. This collection is hereafter cited as SL/UH Collection, MHS.

13. Robb, *Educational Standards*, 224.

14. These totals are based on information from 533 graduates and 293 nongraduates. The specific figures for the nongraduates ranged from .50 years on duty, 1897–1910, to .46 years on duty, 1924–1937. All of the totals include two half days off per week. For source, see table 1. For more detailed information see Thomas Olson, *Women of St. Luke's*, table 11.

15. Conclusions in this paragraph are based on information from the following sources: "Annual Report(s) of Training Schools for Nurses," training program data reported to the New York Board of Nurse Examiners, 1909–1935, Box 1, SLHTS Collection, MHS; and "Annual Reports Required from Registered Training Schools," training program data reported to the Minnesota State Board of Examiners of Nurses Collection (collection also includes surveys and correspondence), 1912–1944, Box 19, MBNE Collection, MHS.

16. Connolly, "Hampton, Nutting, and Rival Gospels," 24, 28. Refer also to the related discussions in the preceding chapters.

17. See previous note regarding source of figures. Note that the figures listed are means. In addition, nurses who had an absence of more than one year (e.g., one woman who "went abroad" for two years) were not included in the totals. The total time in training for nongraduates (including absences and vacations) was, from the first to the last period, .56 years, .64 years, and .68 years.

18. Wendell W. Oderkirk, "'Organize or Perish': The Transformation of Nebraska Nursing Education, 1888–1941" (Ph.D. diss., University of Nebraska, 1988), 216, 278–84. Similar arguments are made by other researchers. See, for example, Philip A. Kalisch and Beatrice J. Kalisch, *The Advance of American Nursing*, 3d ed. (Philadelphia: J. B. Lippincott Company, 1995), chap. 5; Jo Ann Ashley, *Hospitals, Paternalism and the Role of the Nurse* (New York: Teachers College Press, 1976), chap. 3.

19. For nongraduates, 62.2 percent before six months, and 80.6 percent before one year. See previous note regarding source of figures.

20. Lucretia Delaney Himes, interview by author, tape recording, St. Paul, Minn., December 10, 1989.

21. Pat Gaarder and Tracey Baker, *From Stripes to Whites: A History of the Swedish Hospital School of Nursing, 1899–1973* (Minneapolis: Alumnae Association, 1980), 7.

22. Figures cited in this paragraph are from the following sources: "Annual Report(s) of Training Schools for Nurses," 1909–1935, Box 1, SLHTS Collection, MHS; "Annual Reports Required from Registered Training Schools," 1912–1944, Box 19, MNBNE Collection, MHS; and "Annual Report(s) of St. Luke's Hospital," 1892–1920, SL Collection, UHA.

23. Mary M. Roberts, *American Nursing: History and Interpretation* (New York: Macmillan, 1954), 91.

24. Beatrice J. Kalisch and Philip A. Kalisch, "Slaves, Servants, or Saints? An Analysis of the System of Nurse Training in the United States, 1873–1948," *Nursing Forum* 14 (1975): 232.

25. Barbara Melosh, *"The Physician's Hand": Work Culture and Conflict in American Nursing* (Philadelphia: Temple University Press, 1982), 48.

26. Figures cited are from U.S. Department of Labor, Women's Bureau (1932); U.S. Bureau of the Census (1913); U.S. Bureau of the Census (1928).

27. Ibid.

28. These totals are based on information from 806 St. Luke's nurses. Note that a nurse did not begin night duty until she had been in training for at least one month. For source, see table 1. For additional discussion of this issue, as well as a more detailed listing of time spent on the night shift, see Olson, "Apprenticeship and Exploitation," 559–76.

29. For a description of private duty nursing see Bertha Estelle Merrill, *The Trek from Yesterday: A History of Organized Nursing in Minneapolis, 1883–1936* (Minneapolis: By the author [on permanent deposit with MHS], 1944); and Blanche M. Pinkus, "Rolling Along" (a history of the Ramsey County Graduate Nurses' Association), 1938, Minnesota Nurses' Association, Fourth District Collection, MHS. This collection is hereafter cited as MNA/FD Collection.

30. *New York Tribune,* February 18, 1890, 9.

31. "Minutes of the Ramsey County Graduate Nurses' Association," entry from a "special board meeting," January 6, 1926, MNA/FD, MHS.

32. Peter Rachleff, "Turning Points in the Labor Movement: Three Key Conflicts," in *Minnesota in a Century of Change: The State and Its People Since 1900,* ed. Clifford E. Clark Jr. (St. Paul: Minnesota Historical Society Press, 1989), 196.

33. Ibid., 195–222.

34. Ibid.

35. Merrill, *The Trek from Yesterday.*

36. See Kalisch and Kalisch, *Advance of Nursing,* 315–18; and "The Eight-Hour Day," *American Journal of Nursing* 19 (January 1919): 260–61.

37. National League of Nursing Education, *Proceedings of Annual Conventions,* 1912–1950, 184–85.

38. Ibid.

39. "The Eight-Hour Day," 260–61.

40. "Why Join?" *American Journal of Nursing* 36 (October 1930): 1021–22.

41. "Union Membership? No!" *American Journal of Nursing* 38 (May 1938): 573–74. Also see "Nurse Membership in Unions," *American Journal of Nursing* 37 (July 1937): 766–67; and Susan M. Reverby, *Ordered to Care: The Dilemma of American Nursing, 1850–1945* (Cambridge: Cambridge University Press, 1987), 197–98.

42. See Nan Enstad, *Ladies of Labor, Girls of Adventure: Working Women, Popular Culture, and Labor Politics at the Turn of the Twentieth Century* (New York: Columbia University Press, 1999). Enstad argues that working-class women consciously shaped popular culture to dignify themselves as workers and ladies, while middle-class women unfailingly worked to diminish and separate themselves from the lower class.

43. Oderkirk, *Organize or Perish,* 258.

44. Reverby, *Ordered to Care,* 64–65. Also see Kalisch and Kalisch, *Advance of Nursing,* 185.

45. All figures involving practical assignments are drawn from the "monthly records," Boxes 1–5, SLHTS Collection, MHS. For a systematic breakdown of the practical assignments of nongraduates, see Olson, "Apprenticeship and Exploitation," 572.

46. Register of the Sick, 1891–1919, SL/UH Collection, MHS.

47. Ibid.

48. Stewart, *Education of Nurses,* 155–56.

49. Kalisch and Kalisch, *Advance of Nursing,* 184. Also see Roberts, *American Nursing,* 15–16.

50. Conclusions are based on information from the "Superintendents' Report(s)," descriptions of numbers and types of patients admitted to the hospital, 1892–1920, SL Collection, SL/UH Collection, MHS; and the "monthly records," Boxes 1–5, SLHTS Collection, MHS. The remarkable consistency of the assignment records is further highlighted by the fact that the monthly records show that wards closed in response to decreases in numbers of patients admitted.

51. "Annual Report(s) of Training Schools for Nurses," 1909–1935, Box 1, SLHTS Collection, MHS; "Annual Reports Required from Registered Training Schools," 1912–1944, Box 19, MNBNE Collection, MHS.

52. "Announcement," 1901, SL/UH Collection, MHS.

53. "Announcement(s)," 1892–1930, SL/UH Collection, MHS; "Annual Report(s) of Training Schools for Nurses," 1909–1939, Box 1, SLHTS Collection, MHS.

54. Most of the information on courses is drawn from the "Record(s) of Theoretical Work and Examinations," listings of academic work for each trainee, Boxes 1–5, SLHTS Collection, MHS. As suggested, there was a steady increase in the number of women teaching courses. For instance, in 1902 the record of theoretical work and examination shows that thirteen courses were taught by male physicians and only three courses were taught by women. A decade later, the eight initial courses were all taught by women; the remaining courses were taught by fifteen physicians and six women. By 1922, women surpassed men in teaching courses, fourteen to twelve. Most of the women who taught the trainees were nurses, though other female instructors included dietitians, pharmacists, and masseuse.

55. Pinkus, "Rolling Along," 11–12.

56. Ibid.

57. Merrill, *The Trek from Yesterday,* 23–24.

58. Minutes of the Ramsey County Graduate Nurses' Association, 1898–1974, MNA/FD Collection, MHS.

59. Merrill, *The Trek from Yesterday,* 23–24.

60. St. Luke's sought accreditation in 1907. See "Annual Report(s) of Training Schools for Nurses," 1907–1935, Box 1, SLHTS Collection, MHS; and "Annual Reports Required from Registered Training Schools," 1912–1944, Box 19, MNBNE Collection, MHS. Notably, registration and licensure of nurses did not become mandatory in Minnesota until 1960.

61. "Record(s) of Theoretical Work and Examinations," Boxes 1–5, SLHTS Collection, MHS (this record for "M. Wilson," 1912, was the first to list the number of lessons, and thus time, spent in each course).

62. For an example of the irregularities involving course work, see the "Record of Theoretical Work and Examinations," 1916–1919, file "R. Lyons," Box 2, and 1921, "S. Foss," Box 2, SLHTS Collection, MHS.

63. "Annual Report(s) of Training Schools for Nurses," training program data reported to the New York Board of Nurse Examiners, 1909–1935, Box 1, SLHTS Collection, MHS.

64. See for example the 1916 report in the "Annual Reports Required from Registered Training Schools," training program data reported to the Minnesota State Board of Examiners of Nurses Collection (collection also includes surveys and correspondence), 1912–1944, Box 19, MBNE Collection, MHS.

65. On-site inspections took place in 1920, 1924, 1929, and 1934.

66. "Survey of St. Luke's Hospital Training School for Nurses," 1920, Box 19, MNBNE Collection, MHS.

67. Ibid.

68. "Survey of St. Luke's Hospital Training School for Nurses," 1924, 1929, Box 19, MNBNE Collection, MHS.

69. The correspondence between the program and the nursing board reinforces the emphasis on practical training versus academics. It focuses on issues involving individual nurses and questions about "time in training" rather than academic work (SLHTS Collection, MHS).

70. Florence Nightingale, *Notes on Nursing: What It Is and What It Is Not,* 2d ed. (Norwalk, Conn.: Appleton-Century-Crofts, 1860; reprint, New York: Dover Publications, 1969. London: Harrison and Sons, 1860), 127 (page references are to reprint edition).

71. Ibid.

72. "Survey of St. Luke's Hospital Training School for Nurses," 1934, Box 19, MNBNE Collection, MHS. Prior to the 1934 recommendations of the Minnesota Board, the training school committee included the superintendent of the hospital and a member of the alumnae group. In its 1934 recommendation, however, the board argued for the addition of someone "whose *chief* responsibility is the education of the students." The recommendation regarding a director of the school was aimed at the fact that the positions of hospital superintendent and nursing superintendent had been temporarily combined. It is revealing that even the board's language had changed, referring to students, faculty, school, and education, versus nurses, hospital, training, and supervisors.

73. See Committee on the Grading of Nursing Schools, *Nursing Schools Today and Tomorrow, Final Report* (New York: The Committee, 1934).

74. Stewart, *Education of Nurses,* 205–15.

75. In addition to the discrepancies between reporting and reality noted in the text, another issue stands out. It involved the preliminary period, one of the most important plans for academic advancement of early nursing leaders, and an exception to the difficulty in systematically evaluating the emphasis on theory. As initially conceived, the preliminary period was to include six months of academic instruction during which "students were not counted as members of the regular nursing force." The first push to start such a course in the United States came from Mary Adelaide Nutting in 1900. At that time she was the superintendent of the nursing program at Johns Hopkins, one of the most prestigious programs in the country. Nutting contended, "In my judgment the course of instruction for the first year should be so altered as to permit of a certain preliminary training of the pupil before she enters the wards of the Hospital. . . . All necessary study of anatomy and physiology and of materia medica, should form the earliest training and instruction given to a pupil. . . . It would in some measure correspond to the generally accepted methods of teaching in other professions, notably that of medi-

cine" (Helen E. Marshall, *Mary Adelaide Nutting: Pioneer of Modern Nursing* [Baltimore, Md.: Johns Hopkins University Press, 1972], 96–98). Under Nutting's direction, the National League of Nursing Education reinforced the importance of preliminary education in its 1917, Committee on Education, *Standard Curriculum for Schools of Nursing.*

Consistent with the original plan, St. Luke's defined "preliminary work" as a period "with no definite assignment to floors." The training program claimed an eight-week preliminary course by 1909, according to the self-reports submitted to the accrediting agencies. In reality, the record of the nurses' assignments reveals that the preliminary period, as a term focused on academics rather than practical work, did not begin until 1930 ("Annual Reports," 1909–1935). Moreover, until 1924, the preliminary period comprised only zero to .1 percent of the trainees' time in the program. In contrast, vacations and absences constituted considerably larger amounts of time (see Thomas Olson, *Women of St. Luke's,* table 14). The preliminary period was instituted on a regular basis only in the final years of the program, from 1930 to 1935. These are the same years in which entering nurses began taking a semester at the university. During this interval, the preliminary period comprised 10 percent to 15 percent of the nurses' total time in the program.

Yet even this belated change probably did not signal a desire to adopt a more academic focus. Dorothy Slocum, the chief dietitian at St. Luke's in the 1930s and also a member of the "teaching staff" of the program, explains that during the 1930–1935 period "the hospital was in problems." She states the board of trustees was trying to "cut everything— it cost a lot to run the school." At the same time, she adds, a woman was "put in as superintendent of the hospital who was not equipped to do this (Dorothy Slocum interview by author, transcript, St. Paul, Minn., February 15, 1989). In short, there was an obvious economic motivation for shifting some of the initial teaching to the university. As a result of this change, St. Luke's was freed from any financial obligation for the part of the program that reaped the least benefits for the hospital and, from a craft view, a part that was not essential to apprenticeship learning. Prospective nurses simply paid the regular tuition to the university, along with arranging their own room and board for the semester. Upon successful completion of the courses, they began training at the hospital.

76. St. Luke's Correspondence, July 1936, MBNE Collection, MHS; letter to the New York Board of Nurse Examiners, August 24, 1936, Box 1, SLHTS Collection, MHS. Refer also to the related discussion of the program's closing in chapter 8.

Notes to Chapter 5

1. Grace Peter, nee Bakke, interviews by author, tape recording, Willmar, Minn., November 25, 1989, April 1, 1990.

2. Cynthia Q. Woods explains, "Early on nurses contributed their thoughts about the question of professionalism, identifying special knowledge and education as the key. "From Individual Dedication to Social Activism: Historical Development of Nursing Professionalism," in *Nursing History: The State of the Art,* ed. Christopher Maggs (Wolfeboro, N.H.: Croom Helm, 1987), 158.

3. Margaret A. Newman, A. Marilyn Sime, and Sheila A. Corcoran-Perry, "The Focus of the Discipline of Nursing," *Advances in Nursing Science* 14 (September 1991): 1.

4. Joan E. Lynaugh and Claire M. Fagin, "Nursing Comes of Age," *Image* 20 (winter 1988): 184–90.

5. Madeleine Leininger, "Leininger's Theory of Nursing: Cultural Care Diversity and Universality," *Nursing Science Quarterly* 1 (1988): 152.

6. Anne Boykin and Savina O'Bryan Schoenhofer, *Nursing as Caring: A Model for Transforming Practice* (Sudbury, Mass.: Jones and Bartlett, 2001); Madeleine Leininger, ed., *Care: The Essence of Nursing and Health* (Thorofare, N.J.: Slack, 1984); Jean Watson: *Nursing: The Philosophy and Science of Caring* (Boulder: Colorado Associated University Press, 1985); P. Benner and J. Wrubel, *The Primacy of Caring* (Menlo Park, Calif.: Addison-Wesley, 1989).

7. Antonia M. Mangold, "Senior Nursing Students' and Professional Nurses' Perceptions of Effective Caring Behaviors: A Comparative Study," *Journal of Nursing Education* 30 (March 1991): 134–39.

8. M. Patricia Donahue, "Inquiry, Insights, and History: The Spirit of Nursing," *Journal of Professional Nursing* 7 (May–June 1991): 149, citing Isabel Stewart, "The Science and Art of Nursing, Editorial," *Nursing Education Bulletin* 2 (1929): 1.

9. Susan M. Reverby, *Ordered to Care: The Dilemma of American Nursing, 1850–1945* (Cambridge: Cambridge University Press, 1987). Also see Kristen M. Swanson, "Empirical Development of a Middle Range Theory of Caring," *Nursing Research* 40 (May/June 1991): 161–66; and Nori I. Komorita, Kathleen M. Doehring, and Phyllis W. Hircher, "Perceptions of Caring by Nurse Educators," *Journal of Nursing Education* 30 (January 1991): 23–29.

10. Joan Lynaugh, letter to Tom Olson, August 7, 1992.

11. Donna Diers, letter to Tom Olson, March 5, 1992.

12. Suzanne Gordon, "Fear of Caring: The Feminist Paradox," *American Journal of Nursing* 91 (February 1991): 45–48.

13. Lynaugh and Fagin, "Nursing Comes of Age," 184–90.

14. Trudie Knijn and Clare Ungerson, "Introduction: Care Work and Gender in Welfare Regimes," in *Social Politics* 4, no. 3 (fall 1997): 323–24.

15. Nona Y. Glazer, "'Between a Rock and a Hard Place': Women's Professional Organizations in Nursing and Class, Racial, and Ethnic Inequalities," *Gender and Society* 5 (September 1991): 354.

16. Shirlee Passau-Buck, "Caring vs. Curing: The Politics of Health Care," in *Socialization, Sexism, and Stereotyping,* ed. Janet Muff (Prospect Heights, Ill.: Waveland Press, 1982), 203–9. Passau-Buck explains that curing, in contrast to caring, is regarded as stemming from active, masculine traits. She views this as a mistaken idea since "these traits are learned and belong not to one gender but to both" (Passau-Buck, "Caring vs. Curing," 205). Also see Claire Burke Draucker and Anne Burke Lannin, "Willa Cather and the Spirit of Nursing," *Nursing Forum* 27 (July–September 1992): 5; Carol Gilligan, *In a Different Voice* (Cambridge, Mass.: Harvard University Press, 1982); and Evelyn Fox Keller, "Feminism and Science," *Signs* 7 (1982): 589–602.

17. Janice M. Morse, Joan Bottorff, Wendy Neander, and Shirley Solberg, "Comparative Analysis of Conceptualizations and Theories of Caring," *Image: Journal of Nursing Scholarship* 23 (summer 1991): 119–26.

18. Comments on nursing in the St. Luke's Hospital Training School Collection, Minnesota Historical Society, St. Paul, Minn. (hereafter cited as SLHTS Collection,

MHS), are from head nurses, hospital and nursing superintendents, "house mothers" (nursing residence supervisors), and the nurses in training. Interviews with surviving graduates were used to validate and add to this information.

19. "Efficiency Record," 1925, file "V. Iverson," Box 3, SLHTS Collection, MHS. This same approach to titles was emphasized by Grace Peter, nee Bakke, interviews by author, tape recording, Willmar, Minn., November 25, 1989 and April 1, 1990.

20. "Efficiency Record," "Monthly Record," "Record of Nursing Procedures," 1925–1928, file "V. Iverson," Box 3, SLHTS Collection, MHS. It is noteworthy that so many individuals were involved in the evaluation process—with remarkable consistency between individuals in the terminology used—and that there was considerable blurring of boundaries between service and training; comments were as likely to be written by head nurses or superintendents as the instructor.

21. "Record of Nursing Procedures," "Monthly Record," 1923–1926, file "R. Forrest," Box 2, SLHTS Collection, MHS.

22. "Efficiency Record," 1921, "M. Weisbecker," Box 2, SLHTS Collection, MHS.

23. "Efficiency Record," 1921–1924, file "E. Ferrell," Box 2, SLHTS Collection, MHS.

24. "Efficiency Record," 1935, file "I. Kogl," Box 4; and "Efficiency Record," 1936, file "L. Smith," Box 4, SLHTS Collection, MHS.

25. Letter to nurse's sister, February 23, 1932, file "V. Vold," Box 5, SLHTS Collection, MHS.

26. "Affiliation Record," 1929–1930, file "A. Dahl," Box 3, SLHTS Collection, MHS.

27. "Affiliation Record," 1933, file "C. Hines," Box 4, SLHTS Collection, MHS.

28. "Affiliation Record," 1931, file "R. Lee," Box 4; and "Efficiency Record," 1933, file "F. Sittkus," Box 3, SLHTS Collection, MHS.

29. Edythe Berglund, nee Newman, interview by author, tape recording, Phoenix, Ariz., December 30, 1989. Although the interviews are weighted toward the last period, with the earliest interviewee entering training in 1926, this is when the greatest emphasis on academics would be expected, based on the professionalization framework.

30. Virginia Brainard Kunz, *Saint Paul: The First 150 Years* (St. Paul, Minn.: Saint Paul Foundation, 1991), 78–79. See also Paul Maccabee, *John Dillinger Slept Here: A Crooks' Tour of Crime and Corruption in St. Paul, 1920–1936* (St. Paul: Minnesota Historical Society Press, 1995).

31. Grace Peter, nee Bakke, interviews by author, tape recording, Willmar, Minn., November 25, 1989 and April 1, 1990.

32. Ibid.

33. Helen Schendal, nee Bertsche, Scrapbook from nurses' training 1929–1932, Photocopies, St. Paul, Minn.

34. Cited in E. B. Foote, *Advice to a Wife and Mother* (New York: Murray Hill, 1886), 84.

35. "Affiliation Records," 1936–1937, file "C. Cloutier," Box 4; SLHTS Collection, MHS.

36. "Record of Illness," August 8, 1934, file "M. Duitscher," Box 4, SLHTS Collection, MHS. This example is noteworthy, in relation to contemporary nursing, because there is no indication that a physician was consulted prior to carrying out these measures. In current practice, a physician's order generally would be required for a nurse to apply heat and cold. In addition, this example reflects an era that preceded many treatments

and technological advancements that are commonly used today, such as the administration of antibiotics. As a result, nursing work seems to have included more direct,
physical involvement of nurses with patients.

37. "Efficiency Record," 1920, file "G. Rothschild," Box 2, SLHTS Collection, MHS.

38. Jo Ann Ashley, *Hospitals, Paternalism and the Role of the Nurse* (New York:
Teachers College Press, 1976), 84.

39. Reverby, *Ordered to Care*, 51.

40. See for example "Monthly Record," 1918–1921, file "F. Grant," Box 2, SLHTS
Collection"Efficiency Record," 1923, file "G. Clark," Box 2, SLHTS Collection, MHS.

41. Correspondence between nurse and St. Luke's, March 31, 1915 and April 3,
1915, file "L. Smith," Box 5, SLHTS Collection, MHS.

42. Ellen D. Baer, "The Conflictive Social Ideology of American Nursing: 1893, A
Microcosm" (Ph.D. diss., New York University, 1982), 11–12.

43. Judith Godden, "Victorian Influences on the Development of Nursing," in *Scholarship in the Discipline of Nursing*, eds. Genevieve Gray and Rosalie Pratt, 239–254 (New
York: Churchill Livingstone, 1995), 248.

44. Ibid., 249.

45. Ibid.

46. "Efficiency Record," 1921–1924, file "G. Smith," Box 2; "Efficiency Record," 1925,
file "F. Ingram," Box 2; "Efficiency Record," 1928, file "M. Mather," Box 3, SLHTS Collection, MHS.

47. "Record of Nursing Procedures," 1925–1928, file "M. Krch," Box 3, SLHTS Collection.

48. "Efficiency Record," 1922, file "E. Nelson," Box 2, SLHTS Collection, MHS.

49. See, for example, "Record of Nursing Procedures," 1925, file "I. Roberts," Box 3;
"Record of Nursing Procedures," 1926–1929, file "M. Allyn," Box 3; and "Record of
Nursing Procedures," 1925–1928, file "M. Krch," Box 3, SLHTS Collection, MHS.

50. "Record of Nursing Procedures," 1925–1928, file "A. Thompson," Box 3, SLHTS
Collection, MHS.

51. "Efficiency Record," "Record of Nursing Procedures," 1929, file "C. Davies," Box
3, SLHTS Collection, MHS.

52. "Efficiency Record," 1933–1936, file "E. Schutt," Box 4, SLHTS Collection, MHS.

53. "Record of Nursing Procedures," 1928, file "A. Wilson," Box 3, SLHTS Collection, MHS.

54. "Efficiency Record," 1924, file "P. Kongsgard," Box 4; "Efficiency Record,"
1920–1923, file "E. Johnson," Box 2; "Affiliation Record," 1933–1934, file "J. Littrell," Box
4; "Efficiency Record," 1926–1929, file "L. Zopfi," Box 3; "Efficiency Record," 1926, file
"A. Murray," Box 3, SLHTS Collection, MHS.

55. "Record of Nursing Procedures," 1925, file "M. Krch," Box 3; and "Efficiency
Record," 1916–1919, file "L. Abbott," Box 2; SLHTS Collection, MHS; .

56. *Procedures Used in the Teaching of the Principles and Practice of Nursing* (St. Paul:
Children's Hospital, 1930), 24–25.

57. "Efficiency Record," 1927–1930, file "M. Mather," Box 3, SLHTS Collection,
MHS.

58. "Efficiency Record," 1927, file "H. Veen," Box 3; "Record of Nursing Procedures,"
1926, file "P. Cranie," Box 4, SLHTS Collection, MHS.

59. "Efficiency Record," "Monthly Record," 1922, file "E. Swanson," Box 5, SLHTS Collection, MHS.

60. "Efficiency Record," 1932, file "D. Button," Box 4, SLHTS Collection, MHS.

61. These procedures are outlined in two of the texts used by trainees: *Procedures Used;* and Bertha Harmer, *Text-book of the Principles and Practice of Nursing* (New York: Macmillan, 1927).

62. Kathryn McPherson, "Science and Technique: Nurses' Work in a Canadian Hospital," in *Caring and Curing: Historical Perspectives on Women and Healing in Canada,* ed. Dianne Dodd and Deborah Gorham (Ottawa: University of Ottawa Press, 1994), 79–80.

63. It should be recalled that the majority of practicing nurses in the United States do not have baccalaureate degrees, but rather hospital diplomas or associate degrees. Refer again to the preface for a description and notation on the varying entry levels into practice.

64. Refer again to the discussion of this issue in chapter 1.

65. C. Davies and J. Rosser, *Processes of Discrimination: A Study of Women Working in the NHS* (London: Dept. of Health and Social Security, 1986), 55.

66. Ibid.

67. This first definition is from the same article cited previously in describing the typical argument for caring: Mangold, "Effective Caring Behaviors," 134.

68. Jean Watson, *Nursing: Human Science and Human Care* (Norwalk, Conn.: Appleton-Century-Crofts, 1988), 74.

69. Nel Noddings, *Caring: A Feminine Approach to Ethics and Moral Education* (Berkeley: University of California Press, 1984), 30–35.

70. Reverby, *Ordered to Care,* 1. Of course, one could argue that any comparisons between past and present descriptions of caring are invalid, as language changes over time. Clearly, the terms used to describe nursing in the past and present are unlikely to be exactly the same. Yet if there is no resemblance in meaning then current claims to a tradition of caring are left empty. In this regard, Fischer observes that all historical questions are "attempts to establish intelligible relationships between the signs and symbols of our language on the one hand and the evidence of our past on the other" (David Hackett Fischer, *Historian's Fallacies: Toward a Logic of Historical Thought* [New York: Harper Colophon, 1970], 21). Moreover, the work of various researchers underscores the particular importance of attention to language, past and present, in analyses involving gender and work (see, for example, Ava Baron, "Gender and Labor History: Learning from the Past, Looking to the Future," in *Work Engendered: Toward a New History of American Labor,* ed. Ava Baron [Ithaca, N.Y.: Cornell University Press, 1991]; J. Hall, "Disorderly Women: Gender and Labor Militancy in the Appalachian South," *Journal of American History* 73 [1986]: 354–82; and Elizabeth Faue, "The Dynamo of Change: Gender and Solidarity in the American Labour Movement of the 1930s," *Gender and History* 1 [1989]: 138–58).

71. Kathleen Chafey, "Caring Is Not Enough," *N&HC Perspectives on Community* 17 (January/February 1996): 15.

72. Ibid.

73. Ronnie J. Steinberg, "Social Construction of Skill: Gender, Power, and Comparable Worth," *Work and Occupations* 17 (November 1990): 459–60.

74. Ibid.

75. Sam Porter, "The Poverty of Professionalization: A Critical Analysis of Strategies for the Occupational Advancement of Nursing," *Journal of Advanced Nursing* 17 (1992): 723.

76. Luther Christman, "Who Is a Nurse?" *Image: Journal of Nursing Scholarship* 30 (third quarter 1998), 213. Also see Diana Cousin, "Luther Christman Eloquent," *Image: Journal of Nursing Scholarship* 31 (second quarter 1999): 106.

77. Christman, "Who Is a Nurse?," 214. See also Jean Watson, "A Call for Educational Reform: Colorado Nursing Doctorate Model as Exemplar," *Nursing Outlook* 40 (January 1992): 20–26; and Alison L. Kitson, "Johns Hopkins Address: Does Nursing Have a Future," *Image: Journal of Nursing Scholarship* 29 (second quarter 1997): 113. Various other leaders have also called for the doctorate as entry for nursing practice, including Schlotfeldt, de Tornay, Aydelotte, Newman, Carter, and Henry.

78. J. Salvage, *The Politics of Nursing* (London: Heinemann, 1985), 95–101.

79. Linda Norman, "Continuous Improvement in Nursing Education," *IHI Quality Connection* 6 (spring 1997): 4.

80. Cartoon, *Better Homes and Gardens* (September 1997): 256.

81. Celia Davies, *Gender and the Professional Predicament in Nursing* (Philadelphia: Open University Press, 1995), 145.

Notes to Chapter 6

1. Letter to the superintendent, August 1934, file "R. Ortell," Box 5, St. Luke's Hospital Training School Collection, Minnesota Historical Society, St. Paul, Minn. This collection is hereafter cited as SLHTS Collection, MHS.

2. Mary Adelaide Nutting, "The Outlook in Nursing," in *Proceedings of the Twenty-Sixth Annual Convention of the National League of Nursing Education* (Baltimore, Md.: Williams and Wilkins, 1921), 309–10. See also Sandra Beth Lewenson, *Taking Charge: Nursing, Suffrage and Feminism in America, 1873–1920* (New York: Garland Publishing, 1993).

3. Virginia Brainard Kunz, *Saint Paul: The First 150 Years* (St. Paul, Minn.: Saint Paul Foundation, 1991), 70.

4. Bertha Estelle Merrill, *The Trek from Yesterday: A History of Organized Nursing in Minneapolis, 1883–1936* (Minneapolis: By the author [on permanent deposit with MHS], 1944), 76.

5. Letter to St. Luke's, July 9, 1920, file "E. Tanner," Box 5, SLHTS Collection, MHS.

6. Report of the nursing superintendent, 1920, file "E. Tanner," Box 5, SLHTS Collection, MHS.

7. Ibid.

8. Ibid.

9. The specific make up of the Training School Committee was as follows: three graduate nurses; a member of the Board of Trustees; a member of the Medical Board; and the chaplain of the hospital. It considered issues related to the training program, including disciplinary matters. For further information on the committee and its actions, see "Annual Report of Training Schools for Nurses," 1920, Box 1, SLHTS Collection, MHS; "Annual Reports Required from Registered Training Schools," 1920, MBNE Collection, MHS.

10. Letter to St. Luke's and report of the nursing superintendent, July 9, 1920, 1920,

file "E. Tanner," Box 5, SLHTS Collection, MHS. See also W. J. Rorabaugh, *The Craft Apprentice: From Franklin to the Machine Age in America* (New York: Oxford University Press, 1986), 3–15.

11. Philip A. Kalisch and Beatrice J. Kalisch, *The Advance of American Nursing*, 3d ed. (Philadelphia: J. B. Lippincott Company, 1995), 167–69.

12. Wendell W. Oderkirk, "'Organize or Perish': The Transformation of Nebraska Nursing Education, 1888–1941" (Ph.D. diss., University of Nebraska, 1988), ii.

13. Beatrice J. Kalisch and Philip A. Kalisch, "Slaves, Servants, or Saints? An Analysis of the System of Nurse Training in the United States, 1873–1948," *Nursing Forum* 14 (1975): 228.

14. Mary M. Roberts, *American Nursing: History and Interpretation* (New York: Macmillan, 1954), 56.

15. "Efficiency Record," and report of the nursing superintendent, 1920, file "E. Tanner," Box 5, SLHTS Collection, MHS.

16. Report of the nursing superintendent, 1920, file "E. Tanner," Box 5, SLHTS Collection, MHS.

17. "Monthly Record," "Record of Nursing Procedures," and report of the nursing superintendent, 1920, file "E. Tanner," Box 5, SLHTS Collection, MHS.

18. Oderkirk, *Organize or Perish*, ii.

19. Oderkirk claimed a 50 percent attrition rate for those who trained in Nebraska hospitals (Oderkirk, *Organize or Perish*," 306), compared to the attrition rate at St. Luke's of just over one-third (35.7 percent). Indeed, the completion rate of the St. Luke's program (64.3 percent) compares favorably to the current graduation rate of 28 percent for undergraduates attending the University of Minnesota (M. Sandra Reeves and Warren Cohen, "College Guide," *U.S. News and World Report*, October 15, 1990), 124. The graduation rate for St. Luke's is based on information from all 838 women who attended training there, from 1897–1937. For source, see table 1. For more detailed information see Thomas Olson, *Women of St. Luke's*, table 15.

20. Correspondence between nurse and St. Luke's, November 13, 1929, May 7, 1930, file "L. Greene," Box 4, SLHTS Collection, MHS. Miss Greene resigned "because of financial conditions" and her desire to "remain with grandmother . . . as she may not live more than a few months."

21. Wendell W. Oderkirk, "A Peculiar and Valuable Service," *Nebraska History* 80 (summer 1999): 74; also Kalisch and Kalisch, *Advance of Nursing*, 112. See also Jo Ann Ashley, *Hospitals, Paternalism and the Role of the Nurse* (New York: Teachers College Press, 1976), 34–43; and Oderkirk, *Organize or Perish*, 216, 289.

22. Categories and problem rankings were validated by an independent reviewer. A category is listed once per individual, with the result that several related problems may be combined. For instance, the category of "practical work" was listed only once for Miss Tanner, though she had several problems related to practical work. In addition, to avoid providing a skewed picture, no more than three reasons were cited per person (only seven individuals, or 2.3 percent of the nongraduates, had more than three reasons listed). Overall, it was found that nurses who left voluntarily tended to have fewer reasons listed for leaving as compared to those who were dismissed or forced to resign. It should be further noted that while primary reasons were relatively easy to identify, it was not possible to rank the remaining reasons.

23. Letter to nurse's father, September 8, 1924, file "H. Stanger," Box 5, SLHTS Collection, MHS.

24. "Monthly Record," 1924, file "E. Bjerke," Box 4, SLHTS Collection, MHS.

25. Correspondence between St. Luke's, transfer hospital, and the Minnesota Board of Examiners, April 18, 1932, April 19, 1932, April 21, 1932, May 11, 1932, file "F. Quimby," Box 5, SLHTS Collection, MHS.

26. Ibid.

27. Ibid. Similar to this case, it was found that St. Luke's often provided positive recommendations for trainees, even though the nurse had complained about the training program.

28. "Monthly Record," 1927, file "C. Kelly," Box 4; "Monthly Record," 1926, file "S. Balkwill," Box 4; "Monthly Record," 1915, file "G. Peterson," Box 5, SLHTS Collection, MHS.

29. "Monthly Record," 1917–1918, file "H. Bennett," Box 4, SLHTS Collection, MHS.

30. "Monthly Record," 1916, file "W. Montgomery," Box 5, SLHTS Collection, MHS. Another nurse, after "show(ing) signs of discontent," stated that she simply "wished to enter other lines of work" ("Monthly Record," 1911, file "M. Kern," Box 4, SLHTS Collection, MHS). The only situation in which religion was cited involved a woman who resigned after thirty-five days at St. Luke's because she preferred to enter "a Catholic Hospital" ("Monthly Record," 1923, file "M. Wolf," Box 5, SLHTS Collection, MHS).

31. Letter to St. Luke's, ca. September 1910, file "L. Gray," Box 4, SLHTS Collection, MHS. For another similar example see "Monthly Record," 1926–1927, file "E. Havorka," Box 4.

32. Ibid.

33. "Monthly Record," 1921, file "F. Johnson," Box 4, SLHTS Collection, MHS.

34. The explanation for the decrease in this category over time is unclear, though it might be argued that improving conditions, particularly shorter hours, caused fewer women to express dissatisfaction. The data from this category also reinforce the argument from chapter 3 regarding the existence of occupational choices for the nurses.

35. Susan M. Reverby, *Ordered to Care: The Dilemma of American Nursing, 1850–1945* (Cambridge: Cambridge University Press, 1987), 58.

36. Letter to nurse, ca. September 1931, file "A. Hovey," Box 4, SLHTS Collection, MHS. Also see correspondence between St. Luke's, nurse, nurse's family, and affiliating hospital, August 25, 1932, September 2, 1932, November 23, 1932, December 1, 1932, December 6, 1932, December 7, 1932, December 9, 1932, December 17, 1932, January 21, 1933, March 2, 1933, file "B. Heggestad," Box 4, SLHTS Collection, MHS.

37. Ibid. There was obviously some interaction between these areas, although this did not change the distinct ways in which each type of problem was conceptualized and described.

38. "Monthly Record," 1907, file "S. Weitbrecht," Box 5, SLHTS Collection, MHS.

39. "Monthly Record," 1913, file "M. Noer," Box 5, SLHTS Collection, MHS.

40. "Efficiency Record," 1920, file "V. Galloway," Box 4, SLHTS Collection, MHS.

41. Helen Schendal, nee Bertsche, interview by author, transcript, St. Paul, Minn., December 16, 1989.

42. "Monthly Record," 1906, file "F. Hoard," Box 4, SLHTS Collection, MHS.

43. Letters to nurse, nurse's mother, March 23, 1925 and March 25, 1925, file "B. Crossen," Box 4, SLHTS Collection, MHS.

44. Monthly Record," 1921–1922, "B. Balster," Box 4; "Monthly Record," 1909, file "M. Burns," Box 4, SLHTS Collection, MHS. For another example see letter to St. Luke's, September 7, 1933, file "G. Nasvik," Box 5, SLHTS Collection, MHS.

45. For more on this topic see Kenneth M. Ludmerer, *Learning to Heal: The Development of American Medical Education* (Baltimore, Md.: Johns Hopkins University Press, 1995), 77; and Paul Starr, *The Social Transformation of Medicine* (New York: Basic Books, 1982), 135, 138–39.

46. For a detailed listing and discussion of the health of the nurses, see Thomas Olson, "*Women of St. Luke's,* 277–79. Note that nearly three-quarters (73.7 percent) of the trainees reported having two to four "childhood diseases" and one in five had at least one surgical intervention prior to entering the nursing program. Within training, it should be noted that another frequent physical problem of nurses was eczema, linked at the time to harsh disinfecting solutions.

47. Isabel Maitland Stewart, *The Education of Nurses: Historical Foundations and Modern Trends* (New York: Macmillan, 1944), 108.

48. "Monthly Record," 1910, file "B. Kent," Box 4, SLHTS Collection, MHS.

49. Matilda Lindstrom Johnson, reminiscences of her training in 1902, transcript, January 9, 1949, Swedish Hospital Archives, Metropolitan Medical Center, Minneapolis, Minn.

50. Alfred W. Crosby, *America's Forgotten Pandemic: The Influenza of 1918* (New York: Cambridge University Press, 1989).

51. "Close in on Grip," *St. Paul Pioneer Press,* October 11, 1918, sec. 1, 1–2.

52. Ibid. See also Crosby, *Forgotten Pandemic,* 21, 63, 203.

53. Pat Gaarder and Tracey Baker, *From Stripes to Whites: A History of the Swedish Hospital School of Nursing, 1899–1973* (Minneapolis: Alumnae Association, 1980), 13.

54. Merrill, *The Trek from Yesterday,* 51.

55. Ibid., 52.

56. Ibid.

57. Kunz, *Saint Paul,* 69. See also "Grip Fight Grows," *St. Paul Pioneer Press,* November 1, 1918, sec. 1, 1–2.

58. "Influenza Spreads," *St. Paul Pioneer Press,* November 11, 1918, sec. 1, 1–2.

59. E. P. Davis, "Influenza Epidemic," *Journal of Laboratory and Clinical Medicine* (1918): 85–86. Crosby, *Forgotten Pandemic,* notes that individuals most at risk were in the twenty-one- to twenty-nine-year-old age group, a range that included a majority of the St. Luke's nurses in 1918.

60. Letter to St. Luke's, December 19, 1918, file "R. Eaton," Box 4, SLHTS Collection, MHS.

61. "Monthly Record," 1918–1919, file "A. Jasperson," Box 4 (Miss Jasperson developed influenza the same month as Miss Eaton wrote her letter; she died of complications relating to influenza and an appendectomy); "Monthly Record," 1917–1918, file "D. Eggar," Box 4, SLHTS Collection, MHS.

62. Letter to St. Luke's, ca. November 1918, file "F. Edgerton," Box 4, SLHTS Collection, MHS. See also Letter to St. Luke's, October 11, 1918, file "G. Fremow," Box 4; and "Monthly Record," 1918–1919, file "A. Jasperson," Box 4, SLHTS Collection, MHS.

63. Stewart, *Education of Nurses,* 108. In regard to this issue, it is also noteworthy that supervisors responded to nurses who returned to duty after an illness by decreasing the number of night shifts that were required.

64. The shorter work day also may have contributed to the decrease in physical problems, although the eight-hour day was not established at St. Luke's until 1930 (see chapter 4).

65. Thomas Olson, *Women of St. Luke's,* 277–79.

66. Ibid.

67. See, for example, "Physical Examination," 1929, file "B. Palmer," SLHTS Collection, MHS.

68. "Physical Examination," 1925, file "D. Perry," Box 5, SLHTS Collection, MHS.

69. Reverby, *Ordered to Care,* 64; Stewart, *Education of Nurses,* 153–54; Marilyn Givens King, "Conflicting Interests: Professionalization and Apprenticeship in Nursing Education. A Case Study of the Peter Bent Brigham Hospital" (Ph.D. diss., Boston University, 1987), 131; Oderkirk, *Organize or Perish,* 164. The last charge is often connected to the idea that applicants became more scarce with time, a belief challenged in chapter 4.

70. Superintendent's note, ca. 1910, file "N. Howard," Box 4, SLHTS Collection, MHS. For another similar situation see letters to nurses and nurse's sister, February 23, 1932 and June 9, 1932, file "V. Vold," Box 5, SLHTS Collection, MHS.

71. Correspondence between St. Luke's and University of Minnesota Hospital, January 16, 1912, January 22, 1912, February 13, 1912, file "N. Howard," Box 4, SLHTS Collection, MHS.

72. Report of the nursing superintendent, August 1924, file "P. Kongagaard," Box 4, SLHTS Collection, MHS.

73. Ibid.

74. Ibid.

75. Wendell W. Oderkirk, "A Peculiar and Valuable Service," *Nebraska History* 80 (summer 1999): 74. Refer also to the similar discussion and sources earlier in this chapter.

76. Ibid., 76.

77. "Monthly Record," 1922, file "M. Rensch," Box 5; letter to Annie Goodrich, Army School of Nursing, n.d., file "F. Burton," Box 4; "Efficiency Record," 1923, "E. Balfanz," Box 4; "Monthly Record," "Efficiency Record," 1927–1928, file "H. Simonson," Box 5; letter to nurse's father, August 31, 1928, file "G. Aune," Box 4; "Efficiency Record," 1931, file "H. Woodbury," Box 5; and "Monthly Record," 1922, file "E. Swanson," Box 5, SLHTS Collection, MHS.

78. "Monthly Record," 1913, file "R. Richardson," Box 5, SLHTS Collection, MHS.

79. "Monthly Record," 1909, file "I. Stock," Box 5, SLHTS Collection, MHS.

80. Letter to the Superintendent, ca. 1935, and "Monthly Record," 1935, file "C. Lathrop," Box 4, SLHTS Collection, MHS.

81. Interviewees corroborated that "secret marriages" did occur, although they were not common (see Dorothy Slocum, interview by author, transcript, St. Paul, Minn., February 15, 1989; Helen Schendal, nee Bertsche, interview by author, transcript, St. Paul, Minn., December 16, 1989). See also "Monthly Record," 1911, file "V. Spofford," Box 5, SLHTS Collection, MHS.

82. Gaarder and Baker, *Stripes to Whites,* 52.

83. Ibid.

84. Claudia Goldin, *Understanding the Gender Gap: An Economic History of American Women* (New York: Oxford University Press, 1990), 160–66.

85. See related discussions of this issue in chapters 2 and 6.

86. William Osler, *Nurse and Patient* (Baltimore, Md.: John Murphy and Company, 1897), 14.

87. Rima D. Apple, *Mothers and Medicine: A Social History of Infant Feeding, 1890–1950* (Madison: University of Wisconsin Press, 1987), 97.

88. Linda Hughes, "Little Girls Grow Up to Be Wives and Mommies: Nursing as a Stopgap to Marriage," in *Socialization, Sexism, and Stereotyping: Women's Issues in Nursing,* ed. Janet Muff (Prospect Heights, Ill.: Waveland Press, 1982), 158. See also Ronald C. Corwin and Marvin J. Taves, "Nursing and Other Health Professions," in *Handbook of Medical Sociology,* ed. Howard E. Freeman, Sol Levine, and Leo G. Roeder (Englewood Cliffs, N.J.: Prentice-Hall, 1963), 200.

89. Letter to nurse, February 6, 1923, file "M. Webster," Box 5, SLHTS Collection, MHS.

90. Support for leaving to care for relatives is also evident in the following examples: correspondence between St. Luke's, nurse, and nurse's father, December 28, 1926, May 5, 1927, May 16, 1927, file "O. Lawrence," Box 4; and correspondence between St. Luke's and nurse, November 12, 1929, November 13, 1929, November 16, 1929, November 20, 1929, November 26, 1929, May 7, 1930, file "L. Greene," Box 4, SLHTS Collection, MHS.

91. Joan Wallach Scott, *Gender and the Politics of History* (New York: Columbia University Press, 1988), 53–67.

92. Superintendent's note, February 1923, file "M. Webster," Box 5, SLHTS Collection, MHS.

93. Correspondence between St. Luke's and nurse, July 1913 and August 3, 1913, file "C. Clark," Box 4, SLHTS Collection, MHS.

94. Ibid.

95. Letter to superintendent, ca. 1932, file "J. Nelson," Box 5, SLHTS Collection, MHS.

96. Sara M. Evans, *Born for Liberty: A History of Women in America* (New York: Free Press, 1989), 179.

97. It is noteworthy that the percentage of reasons in this category did not increase during the depression and actually decreased from the middle to the last period. Women may have been less likely to return to families during the depression, even to nurse a sick relative, because of the added burden an extra individual would have placed on a family's already strained resources. In the same way, financial conditions may have postponed the decisions of young couples to marry.

98. Superintendent's notes and "Monthly Record," 1922, file "M. Anderson," Box 4, SLHTS Collection, MHS.

99. "Record of Nursing Procedures," "Monthly Record," 1933, "R. Carey," Box 4; "Record of Nursing Procedures," 1924, file "E. Schow," Box 5, SLHTS Collection, MHS.

100. "Monthly Record," 1923, file "E. Torkelson," Box 2, SLHTS Collection, MHS.

101. "Monthly Record," 1921, file "M. Prevey," Box 5; "Efficiency Record," 1930, file

"H. Woodbury," Box 5; and "Efficiency Record," 1929, file "M. Johnson," Box 4; "Monthly Record," 1913, file "E. Reiff," Box 5, SLHTS Collection, MHS.

102. "Monthly Record," 1912, file "E. Dahl," Box 2, SLHTS Collection, MHS.

103. "Monthly Record," 1914, file "M. Pankratz," Box 2, SLHTS Collection, MHS.

104. "Efficiency Record," "Monthly Record," "Record of Nursing Procedures," 1924–1927, file "A. Kruschke, Box 3, SLHTS Collection, MHS.

105. Ibid.

106. "Monthly Record," and letter to employer, 1907, ca. 1909, file "S. Crawford," SLHTS Collection, MHS. "Undesirable personality" constituted 15.8 percent of the total problems included under personality.

107. "Monthly Record," 1922, file "H. Zila," Box 5; SLHTS Collection, MHS.

108. Superintendent's notes, 1919, file "D. Rose," SLHTS Collection, MHS.

109. For additional background, refer to the discussion of this topic in chapter 4.

110. Olson, "Balancing Theory and Practice in Nursing Education: Case Study of an Historic Struggle," *Nursing Outlook* 46 (1998): 268–72; Olson, "Numbers, Narratives, and Nursing History," *Social Science Journal* 37 (January 2000): 137–44.

111. Ibid. Trainees without a high school diploma had a completion rate of 82.67 percent, compared to a completion rate of 64.8 percent for those with a diploma. This difference was significant at the 0.01 level.

112. Barbara Melosh, "Apprenticeship Culture and Nurses' Resistance to Professionalization," in *Alternative Conceptions of Work and Society: Implications for Professional Nursing,* ed. Carol A. Lindeman (Washington, D.C.: American Association of Colleges of Nursing, 1988), 31–54.

113. Letter to St. Luke's, January 16, 1935, file "A. Lefstad," Box 4, SLHTS Collection, MHS.

114. Letter to St. Luke's, November, 1934, file "H. Porter," Box 5, SLHTS Collection, MHS.

115. "Monthly Record," 1923, file "C. Linder," Box 5; SLHTS Collection, MHS.

116. "Monthly Record," 1914, file "H. Nibbe," Box 5; "Monthly Record," 1930, file "C. Ortell," Box 5, SLHTS Collection, MHS.

117. See, for example, Harriet Bradley, *Men's Work, Women's Work: A Sociological History of the Sexual Division of Labour in Employment* (Cambridge, UK: Polity Press, 1989), 194, 632, 684, 672, 823.

118. Ann Game and Rosemary Pringle, *Gender at Work* (Boston: George Allen and Unwin, 1983), 29.

119. Angel Kwolek-Folland, "Gender, Self, and Work in the Life Insurance Industry, 1880–1930," in *Work Engendered: Toward a New History of American Labor,* ed. Ava Baron (Ithaca, N.Y.: Cornell University Press, 1991), 189. See also Barbara F. Reskin, "Bringing the Men Back In: Sex Differentiation and the Devaluation of Women's Work," *Gender and Society* 2 (March 1988): 67–69.

120. Walter Tenerry, a novelist, quoted in Theodore Blegen, *Minnesota: A History of the State* (Minneapolis: University of Minnesota Press, 1975), 205.

121. "Temperance Rally: Twin City Good Templars Hold a Joint Meeting," *Saint Paul Pioneer Press,* March 2, 1897, 3; "To Stop Smoking Among Our Youths," *Saint Paul Pioneer Press,* July 1, 1900, 24; "Wage Purity War on Wickedness," *Saint Paul Pioneer Press,* October 1, 1910, 12.

122. Kunz, *Saint Paul,* 71–73.

123. Ibid., 78–79.

124. George S. Hage, "Evolution and Revolution in the Media: Print and Broadcast Journalism," in *Minnesota in a Century of Change: The State and Its People Since 1900,* ed. Clifford E. Clark Jr. (St. Paul: Minnesota Historical Society Press, 1989), 308.

125. Alvin Karpis with Bill Trent, *The Alvin Karpis Story* (New York: Coward, McCann and Geoghegan, 1971), 100; and Harold Birkeland, *Floyd B. Olson in the First Kidnapping Murder in "Gangster Ridden Minnesota"* (Minneapolis: Author, 1934). See also Paul Maccabee, *John Dillinger Slept Here: A Crook's Tour of Crime and Corruption in St. Paul, 1920–1936* (St. Paul: Minnesota Historical Society Press, 1995); and Steve Thayer, *Saint Mudd* (Washington, D.C.: Pilot Grove Press, 1988).

126. "The Twin Cities are Lousy," *Milwaukee Journal,* September 14, 1933, 4.

127. Minutes, April 4, 1910, Ramsey County Graduate Nurses' Association Collection, MHS.

128. Ibid.

129. Vern L. Bullough, "Nightingale, Nursing and Harassment," *Image* 22 (spring 1990): 4–7; Oderkirk, *Organize or Perish,* 219; Reverby, *Ordered to Care,* 53.

130. Letter to the superintendent, August 1934, file "R. Ortell," Box 5, SLHTS Collection, MHS.

131. A. S. Blumgarten, *A Text Book of Medicine for Students in Schools of Nursing* (New York: Macmillan, 1927), 141–42.

132. "Monthly Record," 1934, file "R. Ortell," Box 5, SLHTS Collection, MHS.

133. Bullough, "Nightingale and Harassment," 4. Bullough's analysis is helpful, although his use of the contemporary term "sexual harassment" to evaluate the past suggests the need for caution in drawing conclusions from his work.

134. Helen Schendal, nee Bertsche, interview by Tom Olson, transcript, St. Paul, Minn., December 16, 1989.

135. Correspondence between nurse, St. Luke's, affiliating hospital, and nurse's mother and sister, February 23, 1933, March 12, 1933, March 16, 1933, March 20, 1933, December 15, 1933, ca. December 1933 (late leave and pass list), December 16, 1933, file "M. Stiteler," Box 5, SLHTS Collection, MHS.

136. Ibid.

137. Ibid.

138. Ibid.

139. Ibid.

140. Correspondence between St. Luke's, nurse, nurse's family members, and "Abortion Release Sheet," March 20, 1933, March 21, 1933, March 24, 1933, December 14, 1933, file "M. Stiteler," SLHTS Collection, MHS.

141. Correspondence between St. Luke's and transfer hospital, June 18, 1935, July 5, 1935, July 10, 1935, July 16, 1935, file "M. Stiteler," Box 5, SLHTS Collection, MHS. It should be noted that various other problems were included under the category of "breaking the rules," such as the following: "continued smoking in her room and other nurses rooms ("Monthly Record," 1929–1930, file "V. Smith, Box 5)"; "conduct with internes [sic}was questionable ("Monthly Record," 1908–1911, file "F. Burton," Box 4)"; "used profanity . . . stayed out late . . . gone to cheap dance hall with two of the maids ("Monthly Record," 1921, file "S. Christenson," Box 4)"; and "returned to Nurses' Resi-

dence intoxicated . . . disobeyed nearly every rule of the School ("Monthly Record," 1928, file "J. Connell," Box 4, SLHTS Collection, MHS)."

Notes to Chapter 7

1. Helen Schendal, nee Bertsche, interview by author, transcript, St. Paul, Minn., December 16, 1989.

2. Ibid.

3. Ibid.

4. Alvin Karpis with Bill Trent, *The Alvin Karpis Story* (New York: Coward, McCann and Geoghegan, 1971), 100. See also Paul Maccabee, *John Dillinger Slept Here: A Crook's Tour of Crime and Corruption in St. Paul, 1920–1936* (St. Paul: Minnesota Historical Society Press, 1995); and Steve Thayer, *Saint Mudd* (Washington, D.C.: Pilot Grove Press, 1988).

5. Helen Schendal, nee Bertsche, interview by author, transcript, St. Paul, Minn., December 16, 1989.

6. Unlike the period before and during training, material regarding the women after leaving St. Luke's was not included in each nurse's file. However, sufficient material was included to provide a picture of nursing after training.

7. "Alumnae Minutes of the St. Luke's Hospital Training School for Nurses," June 12, 1895, St. Luke's/United Hospital Collection, Minnesota Historical Society, St. Paul, Minn. (hereafter cited as "Alumnae Minutes"). Attendance at alumnae association meetings ranged from seven to twenty-five per meeting, with an average of fifteen per meeting. The total number of active (dues-paying) members ranged from the original seven, to forty-nine in 1903, sixty-two in 1915, to sixty-three in 1916.

8. The first local alumnae association of nurses was formed in 1889 by the graduates of the Bellevue Hospital Training School. According to Isabel Stewart, by 1896 alumnae groups "had been formed in practically all the important schools." The same year, the Nurses' Associated Alumnae of the United States and Canada was organized "to consolidate the rank and file (Isabel Maitland Stewart, *The Education of Nurses: Historical Foundations and Modern Trends* [New York: Macmillan, 1944], 139)." In 1911, this organization was renamed the American Nurses' Association, following the withdrawal of Canadian nurses, who formed their own association (see Elizabeth M. Jamieson and Mary F. Sewall, *Trends in Nursing History: Their Relationship to World Events* [Philadelphia: W. B. Saunders, 1950], 438–80). The St. Luke's alumnae group continued to function into the 1950s, although minutes were available only for the period 1895–1916.

9. Mary A. Livermore, "Nurses in the Civil War," in *Proceedings of the Sixth Annual Convention of the Nurses' Associated Alumnae of the United States, June 10–12, 1903* (Philadelphia: J. B. Lippincott, 1903), 1–6.

10. This statement of purpose is similar to that of other alumnae groups, although it is taken from the St. Luke's Alumnae's "Certificate of Incorporation," 1895, SL/UH Collection, MHS.

11. Alan Trachtenberg, *The Incorporation of America: Culture and Society in the Gilded Age* (New York: Hill and Wang, 1982), 217.

12. Philip A. Kalisch and Beatrice J. Kalisch, *The Advance of American Nursing*, 3d ed. (Philadelphia: J. B. Lippincott Company, 1995), 55–56.

13. Susan M. Reverby, *Ordered to Care: The Dilemma of American Nursing, 1850–1945* (Cambridge: Cambridge University Press, 1987), 22.

14. Ibid.

15. Ibid.

16. Frequencies in the table are based on the number of meetings in which an issue was raised. Thus, the total number of times that an issue possibly could be raised equals sixty-three, or the total number of meetings recorded in this time period.

17. "Alumnae Minutes," June 1903, SL Collection, SL/UH Collection, MHS.

18. "Alumnae Minutes," December 1899, SL Collection, SL/UH Collection, MHS, 44. Although members were understandably focused on marriages and deaths of those within their ranks, their concern often transcended their immediate group, such as when they organized to raise funds to decorate and honor the "Wheaton Memorial Room" in honor of a recently deceased St. Luke's physician. An entry in the minutes later noted that this room "is one of the prettiest in the Hospital" ("Alumnae Minutes," November 9, 1915, UH/SL Collection, MHS).

19. An additional work issue addressed by the alumnae involved discussion of the nurses' registry and the "need to accept only nurses from reputable hospital programs." "Alumnae Minutes," December 1910, SL Collection, SL/UH Collection, MHS.

20. "Alumnae Minutes," December 4, 1900, SL/UH Collection, MHS.

21. The insurance plan generally considered to be the nearest prototype of modern hospital insurance systems was not organized until 1929, by the schoolteachers of Dallas. Blue Cross plans subsequently were developed in the 1930s, with a total enrollment of nearly two million individuals by July 1938. Medical insurance lagged behind the hospital plans, which has been largely blamed on the conservatism of the American Medical Association. One exception to this admittedly tardy development of insurance plans was the development in 1880 of hospital-service insurance plans for the benefit of lumbermen in operation in northern Minnesota. See Kalisch and Kalisch, *Advance of Nursing*, 301–5.

22. "Alumnae Minutes," December 4, 1900, SL/UH Collection, MHS.

23. "Alumnae Minutes," June 1913, SL/UH Collection, MHS.

24. Ibid.

25. "Alumnae Minutes," October 1902, SL/UH Collection, MHS.

26. "Alumnae Minutes," April 1908, SL/UH Collection, MHS.

27. "Alumnae Minutes," February 26, 1913, SL/UH Collection, MHS.

28. Lavinia L. Dock and Isabel Maitland Stewart, *A Short History of Nursing* (New York: G. P. Putnam's Sons, 1920), 167–68.

29. "Alumnae Minutes," October 9, 1914, SL/UH Collection, MHS.

30. "Alumnae Minutes," November 9, 1915, SL/UH Collection, MHS.

31. "Alumnae Minutes," December 14, 1915, SL/UH Collection, MHS.

32. "Alumnae Minutes," October 20, 1900, SL/UH Collection, MHS.

33. "Alumnae Minutes," April 30, 1901, SL/UH Collection, MHS.

34. See for example "Alumnae Minutes," September 9, 1903, SL/UH Collection, MHS.

35. "Alumnae Minutes," February 2, 1915, SL/UH Collection, MHS.

36. "Alumnae Minutes," September 15, 1898, June 9, 1907, December 10, 1914, St. Luke's Hospital Training School Collection, Minnesota Historical Society, St. Paul, Minn. This collection is hereafter cited as SLHTS Collection, MHS.

37. Reverby, *Ordered to Care,* 122.

38. These traditions had their roots in the craft guild of Europe. According to Jack C. Ross, *An Assembly of Good Fellows: Voluntary Associations in History* (Westport, Conn.: Greenwood Press, 1976), 141, the central purpose of the guild was originally religious in nature. He adds, however, that this changed over time with the increasing "complexity of the population." Thus, many guilds ceased to "provide a religious organization," while continuing to meet the various other purposes listed.

39. Trudie Knijn and Clare Ungerson, "Introduction: Care Work and Gender in Welfare Regimes," in *Social Politics* 4, no. 3 (fall 1997): 323–24.

40. Blanche M. Pinkus, "Rolling Along" (a history of the Ramsey County Graduate Nurses' Association), 1938, Minnesota Nurses' Association, Fourth District Collection, MHS. This collection is hereafter cited as MNA/FD Collection, 1–2. It should be recalled that the registry was the principal referral agency in the St. Paul area for women doing private duty nursing. See also the discussion of the registry and association in chapter 2.

41. Bertha Estelle Merrill, *The Trek from Yesterday: A History of Organized Nursing in Minneapolis, 1883–1936* (Minneapolis: By the author [on permanent deposit with MHS], 1944), 19.

42. Caroline M. Rankiellour, "The Minnesota State Registered Association," *Minnesota Registered Nurse* 3 (October 1930): 13.

43. Florence Nightingale, "Sick Nursing and Health Nursing," in *Hospitals, Dispensaries, and Nursing, International Congress of Charities, Correction, and Philanthropy, Sec. III, Held in Chicago June 15–17, 1893,* ed. J. S. Billings and H. M. Hurd (Baltimore, Md.: Johns Hopkins Press, 1894), 444–63. This statement is very similar to one made decades earlier by Florence Nightingale, in *Notes on Nursing: What It Is and What It Is Not,* 2d ed. (Norwalk, Conn.: Appleton-Century-Crofts, 1860; reprint, New York: Dover Publications, 1969. London: Harrison and Sons, 1860), 140 (page references are to reprint edition).

44. Stewart, *Education of Nurses,* 136–37; Kalisch and Kalisch, *Advance of Nursing*, 131; Jamieson and Sewall, *Trends in Nursing,* 408; Dock, *Short History,* 161. See also Isabel A. Hampton, "Educational Standards for Nurses," *Trained Nurse and Hospital Review* 10 (1893).

45. Stewart, *Education of Nurses,* 136.

46. "Alumnae Minutes," June 4, 1900, SL/UH Collection, MHS. Note that seventeen members were present at this meeting.

47. "Alumnae Minutes," April 30, 1901, SL/UH Collection, MHS.

48. Merrill, *The Trek from Yesterday,* 26.

49. Ibid., 26.

50. Ibid., 28. See also Stewart, *Education of Nurses,* 139.

51. Ibid., 26–27. The Nurses' Associated Alumnae represented fifteen thousand nurses in 1909.

52. Ibid., 29.

53. "Alumnae Minutes," June 1903, May 1906, SL/UH Collection, MHS.

54. "Alumnae Minutes," January 3, 1914, SL/UH Collection, MHS.

55. "Alumnae Minutes," January 11, 1916, SL/UH Collection, MHS.

56. "Alumnae Minutes," June 16, 1916, SL/UH Collection, MHS.

57. "Alumnae Minutes," April 27, 1908, September 1914, December 14, 1915, SL/UH Collection, MHS.

58. The close ties to other nurses formed by the women of St. Luke's are all the more surprising considering that organized nursing was still in its infancy during the period 1895–1816. In 1880, for example, there were only sixteen training schools nationwide (this number is based on a recount of training schools by Wendell W. Oderkirk, "Setting the Record Straight: A Recount of Late Nineteenth-Century Training Schools," *Journal of Nursing History* 1 [November 1985]: 30–37). In 1900, for every 100,000 people in the United States there were 173 physicians but only sixteen trained nurses. In 1911, while medicine was basking in the glow of the Flexner Report, "a major turning point in American medical education," nursing was more than a decade away from the Goldmark Report (Reverby, *Ordered to Care*, 159, 121; see also Alfred Chase, *The Biological Imperatives* [Baltimore, Md.: Penguin Books, 1973]). Thus, the recency of occupational changes suggested that graduate nurses would be relatively unfamiliar with and involved in broader occupational issues. This makes the St. Luke's findings all the more remarkable.

59. Roslyn L. Feldberg, "Women and Trade Unions: Are We Asking the Right Questions?" in *Hidden Aspects of Women's Work,* ed. Christine Bose et al. (New York: Praeger, 1987), 299–322; Ava Baron, "Gender and Labor History: Learning from the Past, Looking to the Future," in *Work Engendered: Toward a New History of American Labor,* ed. Ava Baron [Ithaca, N.Y.: Cornell University Press, 1991], 1–46; Joan Wallach Scott, *Gender and the Politics of History* (New York: Columbia University Press, 1988), 102–8.

60. Refer also to the discussion of labor organizing and nursing in chapter 4.

61. "Campaign Launched to Organize RNs," *American Nurse* 5, no. 1 (December 1973).

62. Ellen D. Baer, "Nursing's Divided Loyalties: An Historical Case Study," *Nursing Research* 38 (1989): 166–71. See also Nancy Tomes, "'Little World of Our Own': The Pennsylvania Hospital Training School for Nurses, 1895–1907," in *Women and Health in America: Historical Readings,* ed. Judith Walzer Leavitt (Madison: University of Wisconsin Press, 1984), 478.

63. Refer to chapter 3 for a discussion of women's perspectives on the benefits of nursing work and training.

64. Merrill, *The Trek from Yesterday,* 15.

65. Ibid., 13. Refer also to the discussion of private duty nursing in chapter 4.

66. Pinkus, "Rolling Along," 8.

67. United States Department of Commerce and Labor, *Report on the Condition of Woman and Child Wage-Earners in the United States* (Washington, D.C.: Government Printing Office, 1911), 9:24–25.

68. Merrill, *The Trek from Yesterday,* 15.

69. "Trained Nursing," *New York Tribune,* February 18, 1890, 7.

70. Several historians have particularly emphasized the problems of a changing and increasingly crowded job market in nursing. "Beginning after the initial proliferation of training schools," Jo Ann Ashley explains, "nurses were forced to deal with problems of overcrowdedness and competition" (Jo Ann Ashley, *Hospitals, Paternalism and the Role of the Nurse* (New York: Teachers College Press, 1979, 59). However, this was not a problem unique to nursing. As Reverby states, "Other women workers, workers of color, and

the unskilled similarly faced high unemployment, competition for jobs, and lack of collective control over their work" (Susan Reverby, "'Neither for the Drawing Room nor for the Kitchen': Private Duty Nursing in Boston, 1873–1920," in *Women and Health in America: Historical Readings,* ed. Judith Walzer Leavitt [Madison: University of Wisconsin Press, 1984]: 462).

71. La Moure, N.Dak., newspaper article and superintendent's note, n.d., file "F. Brand," Box 1; list of nurses' status after training, ca. 1936, SLHTS Collection, MHS.

72. Correspondence between St. Luke's, nurse, and employer, March 13, 1929, March 18, 1929, October 9, 1932, October 15, 1932, file "D. Benson," Box 1; list of nurses' status after training, ca. 1936, SLHTS Collection, MHS.

73. Leila Halverson, Interview by Lila M. Johnson and Leonora J. Collatz, September 6, 1967, transcript, MHS.

74. Ibid.

75. Ibid.

76. Merrill, *The Trek from Yesterday,* 14.

77. Letter to St. Luke's, August 4, 1934, file "P. Dudrey," Box 3, SLHTS Collection, MHS.

78. Letter to St. Luke's, February 6, 1942, file "E. Rasmus," Box 3, SLHTS Collection, MHS; list of nurses' status after training, ca. 1936, SLHTS Collection, MHS.

79. List of nurses' status after training (D. Lawton and S. Myrah), ca. 1936; note cards listing the status of nurses after training, n.d., Box 1, SLHTS Collection, MHS.

80. Helen Schendal, nee Bertsche, interview by author, transcript, St. Paul, Minn., December 16, 1989. Refer also to the related discussion in chapter 5.

81. Merrill, *The Trek from Yesterday,* 47.

82. Lorraine Brightbill, interview by author, December 9, 1989, transcript, St. Paul, Minn.; Grace Peter, nee Bakke, interview by author and diary recordings, April 1, 1989 and November 25, 1989, tape recordings, Willmar, Minn.

83. Amy Gilman, "'Cogs to the Wheels': The Ideology of Women's Work in Mid-19th-Century Fiction," in *Hidden Aspects of Women's Work,* eds. Christine Bose et al. (New York: Praeger Publishers, 1987), 116–34. Also see Nan Enstad, *Ladies of Labor, Girls of Adventure: Working Women, Popular Culture, and Labor Politics at the Turn of the Twentieth Century* (New York: Columbia University Press, 1999).

84. Letter to St. Luke's, April 14, 1958, file "E. Ryan," Box 3, SLHTS Collection, MHS.

85. Ibid.

86. Letter to St. Luke's, July 10, 1958, file "E. Johannson," Box 3, SLHTS Collection, MHS.

87. See also discussion of family and marriage in chapter 4.

88. Tom Olson, "Recreating Past Separations and the Employment Pattern of Nurses," *Nursing Outlook,* 43 (September/October 1995): 210–14.

89. "Monthly Record," 1928, file "G. Elkan," Box 4, SLHTS Collection, MHS.

90. See, for instance, Nancy Chodorow, *The Reproduction of Mothering* (Berkeley: University of California Press, 1978); Carol Gilligan, *In a Different Voice* (Cambridge, Mass.: Harvard University Press, 1982); and J. Elshtain, *Public Man, Private Woman* (Princeton, N.J.: Princeton University Press, 1981).

91. Baron, "Gender and Labor History," 27. See also Leslie Woodcock Tentler, *Wage-Earning Women: Industrial Work and Family Life in the United States, 1900–1930* (New York: Oxford University Press, 1979).

92. Winifred D. Wandersee, *Women's Work and Family Values, 1920–1940* (Cambridge, Mass.: Harvard University Press, 1981).

93. Louise A.Tilly, and Joan W. Scott, *Women, Work, and Family* (New York: Holt, Rinehart and Winston, 1978).

94. Helen Schendal, nee Bertsche, Scrapbook from nurses' training 1929–1932, photocopies, St. Paul, Minn.

95. The lists of what the nurses did after training were compiled in the 1920s, 1930s, and 1940s by the hospital and the alumnae group (list of nurses' status after training; note cards listing the status of nurses after training, SLHTS Collection, MHS). Refer again to Olson, "Recreating Past," for how this pattern among nurses contrasted with women in teaching.

96. "Monthly Record," 1898–1900, file "I. Dillon," Box 1; list of nurses' status after training, SLHTS Collection, MHS.

97. Donna Diers, "The Art and Craft of Nursing," in *On Nursing: A Literary Celebration,* ed. Margretta Madden Styles and Patricia Moccia (New York: National League for Nursing, 1993), 188.

98. Ibid.

99. Corwin and Taves, *Medical Sociology,* 201. See also Joan E. Lynaugh and Claire M. Fagin, "Nursing Comes of Age," *Image* 20 (winter 1988): 184–90. ; and Lauren S. Aaronson, "A Challenge for Nursing: Re-Viewing a Historic Competition," *Nursing Outlook* 37 (November/December 1989): 274–79.

100. Linda Hughes, "Little Girls Grow Up to Be Wives and Mommies: Nursing as a Stopgap to Marriage," in *Socialization, Sexism, and Stereotyping: Women's Issues in Nursing,* ed. Janet Muff (Prospect Heights, Ill.: Waveland Press, 1982), 160. See also "What Will You Do?" *Trained Nurse and Hospital Review* 107 (November 1941), 367.

101. Scott, *Gender and Politics* citing *La Voix des Femmes* (April 26, 1848; May 30, 1848).

102. Olson, "Recreating Past," 210–14.

103. Ibid. See also United States Public Use Sample, 1940; Claudia Goldin, *Understanding the Gender Gap: An Economic History of American Women* (New York: Oxford University Press, 1990), 13; Regina Markell Morantz-Sanchez, *Sympathy and Science: Women Physicians in American Medicine* (New York: Oxford University Press, 1985).

NOTES TO CHAPTER 8

1. Janet Geister, "Keep the Faith," *Minnesota Registered Nurse* 10 (October 1931): 5.

2. Listing of hospital schools of nursing, 1900–1940, MBNE Collection, MHS. See also Leila Halverson, interview by Lila M. Johnson and Leonora J. Collatz, September 6, 1967, transcript, 20, MHS.

3. Philip A. Kalisch and Beatrice J. Kalisch, *The Advance of American Nursing,* 3d ed. (Philadelphia: J. B. Lippincott Company, 1995), 312

4. Ibid.

5. Letter to nurses' father, January 18, 1935, file "A. Lefstad," Box 4, SLHTS Collection, MHS.

6. Letter to the New York Board of Nurse Examiners, August 24, 1936, Box 1, SLHTS Collection, MHS.

7. Kalisch and Kalisch, *Advance of Nursing,* 3d ed., 312.

8. Halverson interview.

9. Refer again to chapter 4 for a discussion of this issue. Note that the Minnesota Board of Nurse Examiners did not adopt a focus on academic changes until 1934.

10. Florence Nightingale, *Notes on Nursing: What It Is and What It Is Not,* 2d ed. (Norwalk, Conn.: Appleton-Century-Crofts, 1860; reprint, New York: Dover Publications, 1969. London: Harrison and Sons, 1860), 140 (page references are to reprint edition).

11. "A Profession Under Fire," *American Nurse* (May/June 1998): 1.

12. Alison L. Kitson, "Johns Hopkins Address: Does Nursing Have a Future," *Image: Journal of Nursing Scholarship* 29 (second quarter 1997): 113. See "A Profession Under Fire," *American Nurse* (May/June 1998): 1; Pamela G. Reed, "Nursing Reformation: Historical Reflections and Philosophic Foundations," *Nursing Science Quarterly* 13 (April 2000): 129–36; Linda Aitkin, "Transformation of the Nursing Workforce," *Nursing Outlook* 44 (September/October 1995): 201–10; E. Hadley, "Nursing in the Political and Economics Marketplace: Challenges for the 21st Century," *Nursing Outlook* 44 (January/February 1996): 6–10.

13. Kitson, "Johns Hopkins," 115.

14. The dramatic employment shift away from registered nurses toward less skilled nursing personnel is best illustrated by census data. In 1940, for example, the ratio of RNs to all nursing personnel peaked at 73 percent. By 1980, RNs were only 44 percent of all nursing workers, while those in the lowest grade, nursing assistants, grew during the same interval from 9 percent to 41 percent. United States Bureau of the Census, *Sixteenth Census of the United States: 1940* (Washington, D.C.: Government Printing Office, 1943); United States Bureau of the Census, *United States Census of Population: 1980* (Washington, D.C.: Government Printing Office, 1984).

15. Refer to the preface for complete notation on the entry-into-practice debate.

16. Luther Christman, "Who Is a Nurse?" *Image: Journal of Nursing Scholarship* 30 (third quarter 1998): 211.

17. Beverly Henry, "Progress and Prosperity," *Image: Journal of Nursing Scholarship* 29 (first quarter 1997): 2.

18. Kathryn Henley Haugh, "'Nursing by Default': The Evolution of Floor Nursing, 1900–1965," *Windows in Time* 8 (October 2000): 5.

19. Gerard M. Fealy, "The Theory-Practice Relationship in Nursing: The Practitioners' Perspective," *Journal of Advanced Nursing* 30 (January 1999): 79.

20. Ibid.

21. Alice Ream, "Our Undertrained Nurses," *Newsweek* 100 (October 21, 1982): 17.

22. Ibid.

23. Ibid.

24. Ibid.

25. Refer again to chapter 4.

26. Carole A. Anderson, "Social Change and Its Impact on Nursing," *Nursing Outlook* 47 (March/April 1999): 53.

27. Ibid., 54.

28. One of the best-known advocates of doctoral education for entry into nursing practice is Watson, "A Call for Educational Reform," 20–26. Also see Christman, "Who Is a Nurse?"; and Kitson, "Johns Hopkins."

29. Claire M. Fagin and Joan E. Lynaugh, "Reaping the Rewards of Radical Change: A New Agenda for Nursing Education," *Nursing Outlook* 35 (September–October 1992): 213.

30. Barbara Durand, "Quality Research for Quality Practice," in *Communicating Nursing Research Conference Proceedings, Volume 31, Held in Phoenix, AZ, May 7–9, 1998* (Portland, Oreg.: Western Institute of Nursing, 1998), 7.

31. David Powell, "Nurses-Sacrificial Lambs of Healthcare," *RN* 64 (January 2001): 52.

32. Previously cited comments from chapters 2–3.

33. Previously cited comments from chapter 4.

34. Ellen D. Baer, "The Feminist Disdain for Nursing," *The New York Times* (February 23, 1991), A25.

35. Previously cited comments from chapters 3 and 5.

36. Previously cited comment from chapter 4; see also chapter 6.

37. Previously cited comments from chapters 2–3.

38. Previously cited comment from chapter 4.

39. "Editorially Speaking," *Trained Nurse and Hospital Review* 31 (August 1903): 103–4.

40. See, for example, Celia Davies, *Gender and the Professional Predicament in Nursing* (Philadelphia: Open University Press, 1995); Nancy Chodorow, *Feminism and Psychoanalytic Theory* (London: Yale University Press, 1989); Carol Gilligan, *In a Different Voice* (Cambridge, Mass.: Harvard University Press, 1982); Sandra Harding, *The Science Question in Feminism* (Milton Keynes: Open University Press, 1986); Roslyn W. Bologh, *Love or Greatness: Max Weber and Masculine Thinking—A Feminist Inquiry* (London: Unwin Hyman, 1990). Refer also to the discussion of this topic in chapter 3, including the description of the masculine emphasis on knowledge, in contrast to the feminine, as abstract and fixed.

41. Davies, *Gender and the Professional*, 28.

42. Previously cited comment from chapter 3.

43. Phyllis B. Kritek, "Leadership Dimensions in a Human Context," *Nursing Forum* 27 (July–September 1992): 3–4.

44. Previously discussed in chapter 4.

45. Joellen W. Hawkins, "Empowering the New Graduate: A Renewed Professionalism for Nursing," *Journal of Professional Nursing* 8 (September–October 1992): 308; Marlaine C. Smith, "The Distinctiveness of Nursing Knowledge," *Nursing Science Quarterly* 5 (1992): 148–49.

46. Salvage, *Politics of Nursing*, 92.

47. Florence Nightingale, cited in Monica Baly, ed., *As Miss Nightingale Said . . .* (London, Scutari Press, 1991), 95

48. Barbara Melosh, *"The Physician's Hand": Work Culture and Conflict in American Nursing* (Philadelphia: Temple University Press, 1982), 66.

49. D'Antonio makes a similar observation. "We might assume," she remarks, "that marriage, and later, children changed the structure of their (nurses') work: their own domestic responsibilities quite likely precluded the possibility of their spending the sustained days . . . with sick patients. . . . But the well-documented demand that women maintain their nursing role within the socially gendered division of labor suggests the

work itself continued even if its form became more episodic" (Patricia D'Antonio, "Revisiting and Rethinking the Rewriting of Nursing History," *Bulletin of the History of Medicine* 73 (1999): 4.

50. K. Waerness, "On the Rationality of Caring," in *Women and the State,* ed. A. Showstack Sassoon (London: Routledge, 1984), 209.

51. The argument here, like that of Chafey ("Caring Is Not Enough"), is that caring alone cannot explain the richness of nursing, particularly as manifested by average nurses. Refer also to the related discussion in chapter 4.

52. One of the few contemporary nursing theorists to question the goal of nursing professionalization is Kari Martinsen, a Norwegian nurse who argues that practical nursing care is most important in nursing, rather than professionalization and the development of nursing theory. She also states that "the master-apprentice teaching method" is the best way to learn nursing. See Kari Martinsen, *Den Omtenksomme Syke-pleier* (Oslo: Tano, 1993). A summary of her ideas in English is included at the following Internet-based Web site: http://world-nurse.com/theory/kmartin.html.

53. Lavinia L. Dock and Isabel Maitland Stewart, *A Short History of Nursing* (New York: G. P. Putnam's Sons, 1920), 353.

Bibliography

MANUSCRIPTS

St. Luke's Hospital Training School for Nurses Collection, Minnesota Historical Society, St. Paul, Minnesota.

    Accreditation Records and Correspondence, 1909–1935

    Files of Nurses who trained at St. Luke's (graduates and nongraduates), 1897–1937

    "A History of St. Luke's," by unspecified member of the Alumnae Association, ca. 1940

    Note Cards Listing the Status of Nurses after Training, 1892–1937

St. Luke's/United Hospital Collection, Minnesota Historical Society, St. Paul, Minnesota.

    Allopathy and Homeopathy Debate, 1881–1901

    Annual Reports of St. Luke's Hospital, 1881–1920

    Announcements of the Training School, 1892–1930

    Instructions to Women Entering Training, 1892–1930

    List and Descriptions of Superintendents, Managers, Medical Boards, and Matrons, 1892–1937

    List of the Status of Nurses after Training, 1892–1937

    Minutes of the Alumnae Association, 1895–1916

    Minutes of the Board of Trustees, 1891–1902

    Minutes of the Board of Trustees and Managers, 1902–1912

    Minutes of the Ladies' Association, 1882–1891

    Minutes of the Officers and Visitors, 1897–1902

    Superintendents' Reports, 1892–1920

Minnesota Board of Nurse Examiners Collection, Minnesota Historical Society, St. Paul, Minnesota.

    Accreditation Records and Correspondence, St. Luke's, 1912–1944

    Accreditation Records and Correspondence, Various Programs, 1893–1976

    Minnesota Department of Rural Credit Records, Minnesota Historical Society, St. Paul, Minnesota.

    Report Covering System and Operations, 1931

    Minnesota Nurses' Association, Fourth District Collection, Minnesota Historical Society, St. Paul, Minnesota.

    Minutes of the Ramsey County Graduate Nurses' Association, 1898–1974

    Blanche Pinkus's History of the Ramsey County Graduate Nurses' Association ("Rolling Along"), 1938

Swedish Hospital School of Nursing Archives, Metropolitan Medical Center (now Hennepin County Medical Center), Minneapolis, Minnesota.

    Reminiscences of Nurses' Training, 1899–1973.

Interviews and Personal Papers

Edythe Berglund, St. Luke's graduate. Interview by author, December 30, 1989, Phoenix, Arizona, tape recording.

Lorraine Brightbill, St. Luke's graduate. Interview by author, December 9, 1989, St. Paul, Minnesota, transcript.

Leila Halverson. Interview by Lila M. Johnson and Leonora J. Collatz, September 6, 1967, transcript, MHS.

Lucretia Himes, St. Luke's graduate and staff member. Interview by author, December 10, 1989, St. Paul, Minnesota, tape recording.

Christine Nelson, St. Luke's graduate. Correspondence with author, December 20, 1989 and January 15, 1991, Eau Claire, Wisconsin, letters and personal papers.

Grace Peter, St. Luke's graduate. Interview with author and diary recordings, April 1, 1989 and November 25, 1989, Willmar, Minnesota, tape recordings.

Helen Schendal, St. Luke's graduate and staff member. Interview with author, December 16, 1989, St. Paul, Minnesota, transcript and personal papers.

Dorothy Slocum, dietitian and staff member. Interview with author, February 15, 1989, St. Paul, Minnesota, transcript and personal papers.

Dorothy Slocum, dietitian and staff member. Interview by Nancy Johnston Hall, 1987, St. Paul, Minnesota, transcript, United Hospital Archives, St. Paul.

Government Documents

"Department of Women and Children." Minnesota Bureau of Labor, Industries and Commerce. *Twelfth Biennial Report, 1909–1910.* St. Paul: Willwerscheid and Roith, 1910.

Minnesota Bureau of Labor, Commerce and Industry, Woman's Department. *First Biennial Report, 1907–1908.* St. Paul: Willwerscheid and Roith, 1908.

Minnesota Bureau of Labor. *Ninth Biennial Report, 1903–1904.* St. Paul: Willwerscheid and Roith, 1909.

Minnesota. City and County Directories, 1890–1930.

United States Census. Public Use Samples, 1900, 1910, 1940.

United States Census Office. *Eleventh Census of the United States: 1890.* Washington, D.C.: Government Printing Office, 1895c, 1897.

United States Bureau of the Census. *Twelfth Census of the United States, 1900.* Washington, D.C.: Government Printing Office, 1902.

———. *Thirteenth Census of the United States: 1910.* Washington, D.C.: Government Printing Office, 1913a.

———. *Fourteenth Census of the United States: 1920.* Washington, D.C.: Government Printing Office, 1923.

———. *Sixteenth Census of the United States: 1940.* Washington, D.C.: Government Printing Office, 1943.

———. *United States Census of Population: 1980.* Washington, D.C.: Government Printing Office, 1984.

United States Department of Commerce and Labor. *Report on the Condition of Woman and Child Wage-Earners in the United States,* vol. 9. Washington, D.C.: Government Printing Office, 1911.

Books and Articles

"A Profession under Fire." *The American Nurse* (May/June 1998): 1.

Aaronson, Lauren S. "A Challenge for Nursing: Re-Viewing a Historic Competition." *Nursing Outlook* 37 (November/December 1989): 274–79.

Abbott, Andrew. "The Order of Professionalization: An Empirical Analysis." *Work and Occupations* 18 (November 1991): 355–84.

———. *The System of Professions: An Essay on the Division of Expert Labor.* Chicago: University of Chicago Press, 1988.

Acker, Joan. *Doing Comparable Worth: Gender, Class and Pay Equity.* Philadelphia: Temple University Press, 1989.

———. "Hierarchies, Jobs, Bodies: A Theory of Gendered Organizations." *Gender and Society* 4 (June 1990): 139–58.

Aitkin, Linda. "Transformation of the Nursing Workforce." *Nursing Outlook* 44 (January/February 1996): 6–10.

Alexander, Jean H. "Chronological Outline of the Development of Public Education in Minnesota." In *Changing Educational World,* edited by Alvin C. Eurich, 249–57. Minneapolis: University of Minnesota Press, 1931.

Allen, David G. "Professionalism, Occupational Segregation by Gender and Control of Nursing." *Women and Politics* 6 (fall 1986): 1–25.

American Nurses' Association. *A Case for Baccalaureate Preparation in Nursing.* Kansas City, Mo.: The Association, 1979.

"American Troops in France." *St. Paul Pioneer Press,* July 3, 1918, 1.

Anderson, Carole A. "Social Change and Its Impact on Nursing." *Nursing Outlook* 47 (March/April 1999): 53–54.

Anderson, Margo Conk. "Occupational Classification in the United States Census: 1870–1940." *Journal of Interdisciplinary History* 9, no. 1 (1978): 111–30.

Anglin, Linda. "Historical Perspectives: Influences of the Past." In *Nursing Today: Transition and Trends,* edited by JoAnn Zerwekh and Jo Carol Claborn, 31–51. Philadelphia: Saunders, 2000.

Apple, Michael. "Teaching and 'Women's Work.'" *Teachers College Record* 86 (1985): 455–73.

Apple, Rima D. *Mothers and Medicine: A Social History of Infant Feeding, 1890–1950.* Madison: University of Wisconsin Press, 1987.

Arsenault, Elizabeth. "As I See It." *American Nurse* 24 (November–December 1992): 4, 10.

Ashley, Jo Ann. *Hospitals, Paternalism and the Role of the Nurse.* New York: Teachers College Press, 1976.

Austin, Anne S. *A History of Nursing from Ancient to Modern Times-A World View.* 5th ed. New York: G. P. Putnam's Sons, 1962.

Baas, Linda S. "An Analysis of the Writings of Janet Geister and Mary Roberts Regarding the Problems of Private Nursing." *Journal of Professional Nursing* 8 (May–June 1992): 176–83.

Baer, Ellen D. "The Conflictive Social Ideology of American Nursing: 1893, A Microcosm." Ph.D. diss., New York University, 1982.

———. "The Feminist Disdain for Nursing." *New York Times,* February 23, 1991, A25.

————. "Nursing's Divided Loyalties: An Historical Case Study." *Nursing Research* 38 (1989): 166–71.

Baerwald, Thomas J. "Forces at Work on the Landscape." In *Minnesota in a Century of Change: The State and Its People since 1900,* edited by Clifford E. Clark Jr., 19–53. St. Paul: Minnesota Historical Society, 1989.

Baly, Monica, ed. *As Miss Nightingale Said. . . .* London: Scutari Press, 1991.

Baron, Ava. "Gender and Labor History: Learning from the Past, Looking to the Future." In *Work Engendered: Toward a New History of American Labor,* edited by Ava Baron, 1–46. Ithaca, N.Y.: Cornell University Press, 1991.

————. "An 'Other' Side of Gender Antagonism at Work: Men, Boys, and the Remasculinization of Printers' Work, 1830–1920." In *Work Engendered: Toward a New History of American Labor,* edited by Ava Baron, 47–69. Ithaca, N.Y.: Cornell University Press, 1991.

Bayldon, Margaret. "Diploma Schools: The First Century." *RN* 36 (February 1973): 33–48.

Benner, P., and J. Wrubel. *The Primacy of Caring.* Menlo Park, Calif.: Addison-Wesley, 1989.

"Big Buyers Ready to Enter Market, Gotham Bankers Say After Second Crash." *St. Paul Pioneer Press,* October 7, 1929, 1.

Bingham, Marjorie. "Keeping at It: Minnesota Women." In *Minnesota in a Century of Change: The State and Its People since 1900,* edited by Clifford E. Clark Jr., 433–71. St. Paul: Minnesota Historical Society, 1989.

Bingham, Stella. *Ministering Angels.* London: Osprey Publishing, 1979.

Birkeland, Harold. *Floyd B. Olson in the First Kidnapping Murder in "Gangster Ridden Minnesota."* Minneapolis: Author, 1934.

Bledstein, Burton. *The Culture of Professionalism: The Middle Class and the Development of Higher Education in America.* New York: W. W. Norton, 1976.

Blegen, Theodore. *Minnesota: A History of the State.* Minneapolis: University of Minnesota Press, 1975.

Blum, Linda M. *Between Feminism and Labor: The Significance of the Comparable Worth Movement.* Berkeley: University of California Press, 1991.

Blumgarten, A. S. *A Text Book of Medicine for Students in Schools of Nursing.* New York: Macmillan, 1927.

Bologh, Roslyn W. *Love or Greatness: Max Weber and Masculine Thinking—A Feminist Inquiry.* London: Unwin Hyman, 1990.

Bonner, Thomas Neville. *Iconoclast: Abraham Flexner and a Life in Learning.* Baltimore: Johns Hopkins University Press, 2002.

Borchert, John R. "The Network of Urban Centers." In *Minnesota in a Century of Change: The State and Its People since 1900,* edited by Clifford E. Clark Jr., 55–97. St. Paul: Minnesota Historical Society, 1989.

Bose, Christine, Roslyn Feldberg, and Natalie Sokoloff with the Women and Work Research Group, eds. *Hidden Aspects of Women's Work.* New York: Praeger Publishers, 1987.

Boutilier, Beverly. "Helpers or Heroines? The National Council of Women, Nursing, and 'Woman's Work' in Late Victorian Canada." In *Caring and Curing: Historical Perspectives on Women and Healing in Canada,* edited by Dianne Dodd and Deborah Gorham, 17–47. Ottawa: University of Ottawa Press, 1994.

Boykin, Anne, and Savina O'Bryan Schoenhofer. *Nursing as Caring: A Model for Transforming Practice.* Sudbury, Mass.: Jones and Bartlett, 2001.

Bradley, Harriet. *Men's Work, Women's Work: A Sociological History of the Sexual Division of Labour in Employment.* Cambridge, U.K.: Polity Press, 1989.

Brady, Joan. *Fluff My Pillow, Bend My Straw: The Evolution and Undoing of a Nurse.* Long Branch, N.J.: Vista Publishing, 1992.

Bullough, Vern L. "Nightingale, Nursing and Harassment." *Image* 22 (spring 1990): 4–7.

Bullough, Vern L., and Bonnie Bullough. *The Emergence of Modern Nursing.* 2d ed. Toronto: Macmillan Co., 1969.

Burgess, May Ayres. *Nurses, Patients, and Pocketbooks: A Study of the Economics of Nursing.* New York: Committee on the Grading of Nursing Schools, 1928.

Calhoun, Arthur W. *A Social History of the American Family.* Cleveland, 1919.

"Campaign Launched to Organize RNs." *American Nurse* 5 (December 1973).

Cannings, Kathleen, and William Lazonick. "The Development of the Nursing Labor Force in the United States: A Basic Analysis." *International Journal of Health Services* 5 (1975): 185–216.

Carnegie, Mary Elizabeth. *The Path We Tread: Blacks in Nursing, 1854–1984.* Philadelphia: J. B. Lippincott Company, 1986.

Carpenter, Mic. "The Subordination of Nurses in Health Care: Towards a Social Divisions Approach." In *Gender, Work and Medicine: Women and the Medical Division of Labour,* edited by Elianne Riska and Katarina Wegar, 95–130. London: Sage Publications, 1993.

Carr-Saunders, Alexander M., and P. A. Wilson. *The Professions.* Oxford: Clarendon Press, 1933.

Cartoon. *Better Homes and Gardens* (September 1997): 256.

Castle, Henry. *History of St. Paul and Vicinity: A Chronicle of Progress and Narrative Account of the Industries, Institutions and People of the City and Its Tributary Territory.* New York: Lewis Publishing Company, 1912.

Chafey, Kathleen. "Caring Is Not Enough." *N&HC Perspectives on Community* 17 (January/February 1996): 10–15.

Chambers, Clarke A. "Educating for the Future." In *Minnesota in a Century of Change: The State and Its People since 1900,* edited by Clifford E. Clark Jr., 473–506. St. Paul: Minnesota Historical Society Press, 1989.

Chapman, Richard M. "Religious Belief and Behavior." In *Minnesota in a Century of Change: The State and Its People since 1900,* edited by Clifford E. Clark Jr., 507–38. St. Paul: Minnesota Historical Society Press, 1990.

Chase, Alfred. *The Biological Imperatives.* Baltimore: Penguin Books, 1973.

Chaska, Norma L., ed. *The Nursing Profession.* St. Louis: C. V. Mosby Co., 1990.

Chodorow, Nancy. *Feminism and Psychoanalytic Theory.* London: Yale University Press, 1989.

Christie, Jean. "Sarah Christie Steven, Schoolwoman." *Minnesota History* 48 (summer 1983): 245–62.

Christman, Luther. "Who Is a Nurse?" *Image: Journal of Nursing Scholarship* 30 (third quarter 1998): 211–14.

"Close in on Grip." *St. Paul Pioneer Press,* October 11, 1918, 1–2.

Cockburn, Cynthia. *Machinery of Dominance: Women, Men and Technical Knowhow.* London: Pluto Press, 1985.

———. "The Material of Male Power." In *Waged Work: A Reader,* edited by Feminist Review. London: Virago, 1986.

Cohn, Victor. *Sister Kenny: The Woman Who Challenged the Doctors.* Minneapolis: University of Minnesota Press, 1975.

Colvin, Sarah T. *A Rebel in Thought.* New York: Island Press, 1944.

Committee on Education. *Standard Curriculum for Schools of Nursing.* New York: National League for Nursing Education, 1917.

———. *A Curriculum for Schools of Nursing.* New York: National League for Nursing Education, 1927.

———. *A Curriculum Guide for Schools of Nursing.* New York: National League for Nursing Education, 1937.

Committee on the Grading of Nursing Schools. *Nursing Schools Today and Tomorrow, Final Report.* New York: The Committee, 1934.

Committee for the Study of Nursing Education, Josephine Goldmark, secretary. *Nursing and Nursing Education in the United States.* New York: Macmillan Co., 1923.

Connolly, Cynthia A. "Hampton, Nutting, and Rival Gospels at The Johns Hopkins Hospital and Training School for Nurses, 1889–1906." *Image: Journal of Nursing Scholarship* 30 (first quarter 1998): 23–29.

"Corn Reflects Drop in Feeding Operations." *St. Paul Pioneer Press,* February 1, 1931, 13.

Corwin, Ronald C., and Marvin J. Taves. "Nursing and Other Health Professions." In *Handbook of Medical Sociology,* edited by Howard E. Freeman, Sol Levine, and Leo G. Roeder, 187–212. Englewood Cliffs, N.J.: Prentice-Hall, 1963.

Cory, Margaret Heyse. *Nurse: A Changing Word in A Changing World: The History of the University of North Dakota College of Nursing, 1909–1982.* Grand Forks, N.Dak.: University Press, 1982.

Coulter, Harris L. *Divided Legacy: The Conflict Between Homeopathy and the American Medical Association: Science and Ethics in American Medicine, 1800–1900,* vol. 3. 2d ed. Berkeley: North Atlantic Press, 1988.

Council on Medical Education and Hospitals of the American Medical Association. "Third Presentation of Hospital Data." *Journal of the American Medical Association* 82 (1924): 118.

Cousin, Diana. "Luther Christman Eloquent." *Image: Journal of Nursing Scholarship* 31 (second quarter 1999): 106.

Crompton, Rosemary, and Kay Sanderson. *Gendered Jobs and Social Change.* London: Unwin Hyman, 1990.

"Crops Excellent, Reports Indicate." *St. Paul Pioneer Press,* July 7, 1918, 2.

Crosby, Alfred W. *America's Forgotten Pandemic: The Influenza of 1918.* New York: Cambridge University Press, 1989.

D'Antonio, Patricia. "Rethinking the Rewriting of Nursing History." *Chronicle* 9 (spring 1998): 3–4.

———. "Revisiting and Rethinking the Rewriting of Nursing History." *Bulletin of the History of Medicine* 73 (1999): 268–90.

Daniels, Arlene Kaplan. "Invisible Work." *Social Problems* 34 (1987): 403–13.

Davies, Celia. *Gender and the Professional Predicament in Nursing.* Philadelphia: Open University Press, 1995.

———. "Professional Power and Sociological Analysis: Lessons from a Comparative Historical Study of Nursing in Britain and the U.S.A." Ph.D. diss., University of Warwick, 1981.

Davies, C., and J. Rosser. *Processes of Discrimination: A Study of Women Working in the NHS.* London: Dept. of Health and Social Security, 1986.

Davis, E. P. "Influenza Epidemic." *Journal of Laboratory and Clinical Medicine* (1918): 85–86.

DeVault, Ileen A. "'Give the Boys a Trade': Gender and Job Choice in the 1890s." In *Work Engendered: Toward a New History of American Labor,* edited by Ava Baron, 191–215. Ithaca, N.Y.: Cornell University Press, 1991.

Diers, Donna. "The Art and Craft of Nursing." In *On Nursing: A Literary Celebration,* ed. Margretta Madden Styles and Patricia Moccia, 186–88. New York: National League for Nursing, 1993.

Dock, Lavinia L., and Isabel Maitland Stewart. *A Short History of Nursing.* New York: G. P. Putnam's Sons, 1920.

Dolan, Josephine A., M. Louise Fitzpatrick, and Eleanor Krohn Herrmann. *Nursing in Society: A Historical Perspective.* 15th ed. Philadelphia: W. B. Saunders Co., 1983.

Donahue, M. Patricia. "Inquiry, Insight, and History: The Spirit of Nursing." *Journal of Professional Nursing* 7 (May–June 1991): 149.

Draucker, Claire Burke, and Anne Burke Lannin. "Willa Cather and the Spirit of Nursing." *Nursing Forum* 27 (July–September 1992): 5–11.

Durand, Barbara. "Quality Research for Quality Practice." In *Communicating Nursing Research Conference Proceedings, Volume 31, Held in Phoenix, AZ, May 7–9, 1998,* 3–15. Portland, Ore.: Western Institute of Nursing, 1998.

"Editorially Speaking." *Trained Nurse and Hospital Review* 31 (August 1903): 103–4.

Eggleston, Edward. *The Mystery of Metropolisville.* New York: Orange Judd and Co., 1873.

"The Eight-Hour Day." *American Journal of Nursing* 19 (January 1919): 260–61.

Ellis, Janice Rider, and Celia Love Hartley. *Nursing in Today's World: Challenges, Issues, and Trends.* Philadelphia: Lippincott, 2001.

Enstad, Nan. *Ladies of Labor, Girls of Adventure: Working Women, Popular Culture, and Labor Politics at the Turn of the Twentieth Century.* New York: Columbia University Press, 1999.

Etzioni, Amitai. *Modern Organizations.* Englewood Cliffs, N.J.: Prentice-Hall, 1964.

Evans, Sara M. *Born for Liberty: A History of Women in America.* New York: Free Press, 1989.

Fagin, Claire M., and Joan E. Lynaugh. "Reaping the Rewards of Radical Change: A New Agenda for Nursing Education." *Nursing Outlook* 35 (September–October 1992): 213–220.

Faue, Elizabeth. "The Dynamo of Change: Gender and Solidarity in the American Labour Movement of the 1930's." *Gender and History* 1 (summer 1989): 138–58.

Fealy, Gerard M. "The Theory-Practice Relationship in Nursing: The Practitioners' Perspective." *Journal of Advanced Nursing* 30 (January 1999): 74–82.

Feldberg, Roslyn L. "Women and Trade Unions: Are We Asking the Right Questions?" In *Hidden Aspects of Women's Work,* edited by Christine Bose et al., 299–322. New York: Praeger, 1987.

Fischer, David Hackett. *Historians Fallacies: Toward a Logic of Historical Thought.* New York: Harper Colophon Books, 1970.

Fitzpatrick, M. Louise. "A Historical Study of Nursing Organization: Doing Historical Research." In *Nursing Research: A Qualitative Perspective,* edited by P. L. Munhall and Carolyn J. Oiler, 195–225. Norwalk, Conn.: Appleton-Century- Crofts, 1986.

———. *Prologue to Professionalism.* Bowie, Md.: Robert J. G. Brady Co., 1983.

Flexner, Abraham. "Is Social Work a Profession?" *Proceedings of the National Conference of Charities and Correction,* 576–90. Chicago: Hildman Printing Co., 1915.

———. *Medical Education in the United States and Canada: A Report to the Carnegie Foundation for the Advancement of Teaching.* New York: Carnegie Foundation for the Advancement of Teaching, 1910; reprint, New York: Arno Press and the New York Times, 1972.

Folwell, William Watts. *A History of Minnesota,* vol. 3. St. Paul: Minnesota Historical Society, 1969.

Fondiller, S. H. "The Entry Issue: How Much Longer? An Historian's View." *Journal of the New York State Nurses Association* 17 (June 1986): 7–14.

Foote, E. G. *Advice to a Wife and Mother.* New York: Murray Hill, 1886.

Freidson, Eliot. *Professional Powers: A Study of the Institutionalization of Formal Knowledge.* Chicago: University of Chicago Press, 1986.

Frohnmayer, John L. "The Captive Conscience: Teaching in an Age of Intellectual Intimidation." *National Teaching and Learning Forum* 7 (1998): 6.

Gamble, Vanessa Northington. *Making a Place for Ourselves: The Black Hospital Movement, 1920–1945.* New York: Oxford University Press, 1995.

Game, Ann, and Rosemary Pringle. *Gender at Work.* Boston: George Allen and Unwin, 1983.

Garling, Jean. "Flexner and Goldmark: Why the Difference in Impact." *Nursing Outlook* 33 (January/February 1985): 26–31.

Gaarder, Pat, and Tracey Baker. *From Stripes to Whites: A History of the Swedish Hospital School of Nursing, 1899–1973.* Minneapolis: Alumnae Association, 1980.

Geister, Janet. "Keep the Faith." *The Minnesota Registered Nurse* 10 (October 1931): 5.

Gilligan, Carol. *In a Different Voice: Psychological Theory and Women's Development.* Boston: Harvard University Press, 1982.

Gilman, Amy. "'Cogs to the Wheels': The Ideology of Women's Work in Mid-19th-Century Fiction." In *Hidden Aspects of Women's Work,* edited by Christine Bose et al., 116–34. New York: Praeger, 1987.

Glantz, Stanton A. *Primer of Biostatistics.* New York: McGraw-Hill, 1992.

Glazer, Nona Y. "'Between a Rock and a Hard Place': Women's Professional Organizations in Nursing and Class, Racial, and Ethnic Inequalities." *Gender and Society* 5 (September 1991): 351–72.

Glazer, P., and M. Slater. *Unequal Colleagues: The Entrance Of Women into the Professions, 1890–1940.* New Brunswick: Rutgers University Press, 1987.

Godden, Judith. "Nightingale's Legacy and Hours of Work." In *Nursing History and the Politics of Welfare,* edited by Anne Marie Rafferty, Jane Robinson, and Ruth Elkan. New York: Routledge, 1997.

———. "Victorian Influences on the Development of Nursing." In *Scholarship in the Discipline of Nursing,* edited by Genevieve Gray and Rosalie Pratt, 239–54. New York: Churchill Livingstone, 1995.

Goldin, Claudia. *Understanding the Gender Gap: An Economic History of American Women.* New York: Oxford University Press, 1990.

Gordon, Suzanne. "Fear of Caring: The Feminist Paradox." *American Journal of Nursing* 91 (February 1991): 45–48.

Grando, Victoria T. "Class Status among Student Nurses at the University of Kansas School of Nursing, 1907–1929." Paper presented at the Eighth Annual Conference on Nursing History, San Francisco, September 28–29, 1991.

Gray, James. *Education for Nursing: A History of the University of Minnesota School.* Minneapolis: University of Minnesota Press, 1960.

"Grip Fight Grows." *St. Paul Pioneer Press*, November 1, 1918, 1–2.

Groneman, Carol, and Mary Beth Norton, eds. *"To Toil the Livelong Day": America's Women at Work, 1780–1980.* Ithaca, N.Y.: Cornell University Press, 1987.

"Guard Closes Blooming Prairie Bars." *St. Paul Pioneer Press*, July 2, 1918, 1.

Hage, George S. "Evolution and Revolution in the Media: Print and Broadcast Journalism." In *Minnesota in a Century of Change: The State and Its People since 1900*, edited by Clifford E. Clark Jr., 295–328. St. Paul: Minnesota Historical Society, 1989.

Hall, J. D. "Disorderly Women: Gender and Labor Militancy in the Appalachian South." *Journal of American History* 73 (1986): 354–82.

Hall, Nancy Johnston, and Mary Bround Smith. *Traditions United: The History of St. Luke's and Charles T. Miller Hospitals and Their Service to St. Paul.* St. Paul: United Hospital Foundation, 1987.

Halloran, Edward J. "Men in Nursing." In *Current Issues in Nursing*, edited by Joanne Comi McCloskey and Helen Kennedy Grace, 969–78. Boston: Blackwell Scientific Publications, 1985.

Hampton, Isabel. *Educational Standards for Nurses.* Cleveland: E. C. Koeckert, 1907.

Hampton, Isabel A. "Educational Standards for Nurses." *Trained Nurse and Hospital Review* 10 (1893).

———. "Educational Standards for Nurses." In *Nursing of the Sick (papers presented at the International Congress of Charities, Correction, and Philanthropy) Held in Chicago, 1893*, 1–12. New York: McGraw-Hill, 1893.

Harding, Sandra. *The Science Question in Feminism.* Milton Keynes: Open University Press, 1986.

Hardy, Evelyn. "Letters." *American Journal of Nursing* 60 (December 1960): 1702.

Hare-Mustin, R., and J. Marecek, eds. *Making a Difference: Psychology and the Construction of Gender.* New Haven, Conn.: Yale University Press, 1990.

Harmer, Bertha. *Text-book of the Principles and Practice of Nursing.* New York: Macmillan, 1927.

Harris, Chauncy D. "Agricultural Production in the United States: The Last Fifty Years and the Next." *Geographical Review* 60 (1970): 50–51.

Haugh, Kathryn Henley. "'Nursing by Default': The Evolution of Floor Nursing, 1900–1965." *Windows in Time* 8 (October 2000): 5–7.

Hawkins, Joellen W. "Empowering the New Graduate: A Renewed Professionalism for Nursing." *Journal of Professional Nursing* 8 (September–October 1992): 308–12.

Henry, Beverly. "Progress and Prosperity." *Image: Journal of Nursing Scholarship* 29 (first quarter 1997): 2.

214 *Bibliography*

Hine, Darlene Clark. *Black Women in White: Racial Conflict Cooperation in the Nursing Profession, 1890–1950.* Bloomington: Indiana University Press, 1989.

Hiraki, Akemi. "Tradition, Rationality, and Power in Introductory Nursing Textbooks: A Critical Hermeneutics Study." *Advances in Nursing Science* 14 (March 1992): 1–12.

Hobsbawm, Eric. *Workers: Worlds of Labor.* New York: Pantheon Books, 1984.

Holmquist, June Drenning, ed. *They Chose Minnesota: A Survey of the State's Ethnic Groups.* St. Paul: Minnesota Historical Society Press, 1981.

Horton, Sandra. "Feminine Authority and Social Order: Florence Nightingale's Conception of Nursing and Health Care." *Social Analysis* 15 (1984): 59–101.

Houlton, R. *The Profession of Nursing.* Minneapolis: Woman's Occupational Bureau, 1930.

Hughes, Linda. "Little Girls Grow Up to Be Wives and Mommies: Nursing as a Stopgap to Marriage." In *Socialization, Sexism, and Stereotyping: Women's Issues in Nursing,* edited by Janet Muff, 157–168. Prospect Heights, Ill.: Waveland Press, 1982.

"Influenza Spreads." *St. Paul Pioneer Press,* November 11, 1918, 1–2.

Irigaray, Luce. *Je, Tu, Vous: Toward a Culture of Difference.* London: Routledge, 1993.

"Italians Gain Advantage by Surprise Onslaught." *St. Paul Pioneer Press,* July 1, 1918, 1.

James, Janet Wilson. "Isabel Hampton and the Professionalization of Nursing." In *The Therapeutic Revolution: Essays in the Social History of American Medicine,* edited by M. J. Vogel and C. E. Rosenberg, 201–44. Philadelphia: University of Pennsylvania Press, 1979.

———. "Writing and Rewriting Nursing History: A Review Essay." *Bulletin of the History of Medicine* 58 (1984): 568.

Jamieson, Elizabeth M., and Mary F. Sewall. *Trends in Nursing History: Their Relationship to World Events.* Philadelphia: W. B. Saunders, 1950.

Jeffrey, Kirk. "The Major Manufacturers: From Food and Forest Products to High Technology." In *Minnesota in a Century of Change: The State and Its People Since 1900,* edited by Clifford E. Clark Jr., 223–59. St. Paul: Minnesota Historical Society, 1989.

Jelatis, Virginia. "The Measurement of Changing Occupational Structure in Public Use Samples, 1880–1980." Paper presented at the Fifteenth Annual Meeting of the Social Science History Association, Minneapolis, Minnesota, October 18–21, 1990.

Jones, Kathleen B. *Compassionate Authority: Democracy and the Representation of Women.* London: Routledge, 1993.

Joslin, Florence M. "The Ideal Nurse." *Trained Nurse and Hospital Review* 52 (January 1914): 44.

Kalisch, Philip A., and Beatrice J. Kalisch. *The Advance of American Nursing.* 2d ed. Boston: Little, Brown and Co., 1986.

———. *The Advance of American Nursing.* 3d ed. Philadelphia: J. B. Lippincott Company, 1995.

———. "Slaves, Servants, or Saints? An Analysis of the System of Nurse Training in the United States, 1873–1948." *Nursing Forum* 14 (1975): 223–63.

Karpis, Alvin, with Bill Trent. *The Alvin Karpis Story.* New York: Coward, McCann and Geoghegan, 1971.

Katznelson, Ira. "Working-Class Formation: Constructing Cases and Comparisons." In *Working-Class Formation: Nineteenth-Century Patterns in Western Europe and the*

United States, edited by Ira Katznelson and Aristide R. Zolberg, 3–41. Princeton, N.J.: Princeton University Press, 1986.

Kaufman, Martin. *Homeopathy in America: The Rise and Fall of a Medical Heresy.* Baltimore: Johns Hopkins Press, 1971.

Keillor, Garrison. *Lake Wobegon Days.* New York: Penguin, 1995.

Keller, Evelyn Fox. "Feminism and Science." *Signs* 7 (1982): 589–602.

Kessler-Harris, Alice. *Women Have Always Worked: A Historical Overview.* New York: Feminist Press, 1981.

King, Marilyn Givens. "Conflicting Interests: Professionalization and Apprenticeship in Nursing Education. A Case Study of the Peter Bent Brigham Hospital." Ph.D. diss., Boston University, 1987.

Kitson, Alison L. "Johns Hopkins Address: Does Nursing Have a Future?" *Image: Journal of Nursing Scholarship* 29 (second quarter 1997): 111–15.

Knijn, Trudie, and Clare Ungerson. "Introduction: Care Work and Gender in Welfare Regimes." *Social Politics* 4, no. 3 (fall 1997): 323–27.

Koerner, JoEllen. "Differentiated Practice: The Evolution of Professional Nursing." *Journal of Professional Nursing* 8 (November–December 1992): 335–41.

Komorita, Nori I., Kathleen M. Doehring, and Phyllis W. Hircher. "Perceptions of Caring by Nurse Educators." *Journal of Nursing Education* 30 (January 1991): 23–29.

Kritek, Phyllis B. "Leadership Dimensions in a Human Context." *Nursing Forum* 27 (July–September 1992): 3–4.

Kunz, Virginia Brainard. *Saint Paul: The First 150 Years.* St. Paul: Saint Paul Foundation, 1991.

Kwolek-Folland, Angel. "Gender, Self, and Work in the Life Insurance Industry, 1880–1930." In *Work Engendered: Toward a New History of American Labor,* edited by Ava Baron, 168–90. Ithaca, N.Y.: Cornell University Press, 1991.

Larsen, Arthur J., ed. *Crusader and Feminist: Letters of Jane Grey Swisshelm, 1858–1865.* St. Paul: Minnesota Historical Society, 1934.

Larson, Magali S. *The Rise of Professionalism: A Sociological Analysis.* Berkeley: University of California Press, 1977.

Laurie, Bruce. *Artisans into Workers: Labor in Nineteenth-Century America.* New York: Hill and Wang, 1989.

Lehrer, Susan. "A Living Wage Is for Men Only: Minimum Wage Legislation for Women, 1910–1925." In *Hidden Aspects of Women's Work,* edited by Christine Bose et al. New York: Praeger, 1987.

Leighhow, Susan Rimby. "Backrubs vs. Bach: Nursing and the Entry-into-Practice Debate, 1946–1986." *Nursing History Review* 4 (1996): 3–17.

Leininger, Madeleine, ed. *Care: The Essence of Nursing and Health.* Thorofare, N.J.: Slack, 1984.

———. "Leininger's Theory of Nursing: Cultural Care Diversity and Universality." *Nursing Science Quarterly* 1 (1988): 152–60.

Lewenson, Sandra Beth. *Taking Charge: Nursing, Suffrage and Feminism in America, 1873–1920.* New York: Garland Publishing, 1993.

Lewis, Sinclair. *Main Street.* New York: Harcourt, Brace and Howe, 1920.

Livermore, Mary A. "Nurses in the Civil War." In *Proceedings of the Sixth Annual Convention of the Nurses' Associated Alumnae of the United States, June 10–12, 1903,* 1–6. Philadelphia: J. B. Lippincott, 1903.

Ludmerer, Kenneth M. *Learning to Heal: The Development of American Medical Education.* Baltimore: Johns Hopkins University Press, 1995.

———. *Time to Heal: American Medical Education from the Turn of the Century to the Era of Managed Care.* New York: Oxford University Press, 1999.

Lynaugh, Joan E. "Narrow Passageways: Nurses and Physicians in Conflict and Concert Since 1875." In *The Physician as Captain of the Ship: A Critical Reappraisal,* edited by Nancy M. P. King, Larry R. Churchill, and Alan W. Cross, 23–37. Boston: D. Reidel Publishing, 1988.

———. "From Respectable Domesticity to Medical Efficiency: The Changing Kansas City Hospital, 1875–1920." In *The American Hospital: Communities and Social Contexts,* edited by Diana Elizabeth Long and Janet Golden, 21–39. Ithaca, N.Y.: Cornell University Press, 1989.

Lynaugh, Joan E., and Claire M. Fagin. "Nursing Comes of Age." *Image* 20 (winter 1988): 184–90.

Maccabee, Paul. *John Dillinger Slept Here: A Crooks' Tour of Crime and Corruption in St. Paul, 1920–1936.* St. Paul: Minnesota Historical Society Press, 1995.

Mangold, Antonia M. "Senior Nursing Students' and Professional Nurses' Perceptions of Effective Caring Behaviors: A Comparative Study." *Journal of Nursing Education* 30 (March 1991): 134–39.

Marshall, Elaine Sorensen, and Barbra Mann Wall. "Religion, Gender, and Autonomy: A Comparison of Two Religious Women's Groups in Nursing and Hospitals in the Late Nineteenth and Early Twentieth Centuries." *Advances in Nursing Science* 22 (1999): 1–22.

Marshall, Helen E. *Mary Adelaide Nutting: Pioneer of Modern Nursing.* Baltimore: Johns Hopkins University Press, 1972.

Martin, Molly, ed. *Hard-Hatted Women: Stories of Struggle and Success in the Trades.* Seattle: Seal Press, 1988.

Martinson, Kari. *Den Omtenksomme Sykepleier.* Oslo: Tano, 1993 (http://world-nurse.com/theory/kmartin.html).

McPherson, Kathryn. "Science and Technique: Nurses' Work in a Canadian Hospital." In *Caring and Curing: Historical Perspectives on Women and Healing in Canada,* edited by Dianne Dodd and Deborah Gorham, 71–101. Ottawa: University of Ottawa Press, 1994.

Meier, Peg. "When Sister Kenny Came to Minneapolis." *Minneapolis Star Tribune,* December 17, 1992, sec. E, 1–3.

Melosh, Barbara. "Apprenticeship Culture and Nurses' Resistance to Professionalization." In *Alternative Conceptions of Work and Society: Implications for Professional Nursing,* edited by Carol A. Lindeman, 31–54. Washington, D.C.: American Association of Colleges of Nursing, 1988.

———. *"The Physician's Hand": Work Culture and Conflict in American Nursing.* Philadelphia: Temple University Press, 1982.

Merrill, Bertha Etelle. *The Trek from Yesterday: A History of Organized Nursing in Minneapolis, 1883–1936.* Minneapolis: Author, 1944 (on permanent deposit with the Minnesota Historical Society).

Meyer, R. "Letters." *American Journal of Nursing* 62 (August 1962): 16.

Milkman, Ruth, ed. *Women, Work and Protest.* Boston: Routledge and Kegan Paul, 1985.

Mills, Albert J., and Peta Tancred, eds. *Gendering Organizational Analysis.* London: Sage, 1992.

Montgomery, David. *The Fall of the House of Labor: The Workplace, the State, and American Labor Activism, 1865–1925.* New York: Cambridge University Press, 1987.

Moore, Judith. *A Zeal for Responsibility: The Struggle for Professional Nursing in Victorian England, 1868–1883.* Athens: University of Georgia, 1988.

Morantz-Sanchez, Regina Markell. *Sympathy and Science: Women Physicians in American Medicine.* New York: Oxford University Press, 1985.

Morse, Janice M., Joan Bottorff, Wendy Neander, and Shirley Solberg. "Comparative Analysis of Conceptualizations and Theories of Caring." *Image: Journal of Nursing Scholarship* 23 (summer 1991): 119–26.

"Mothers Here Lack Patriotism." *St. Paul Pioneer Press,* July 10, 1918, 5.

Mottus, Jane E. *New York Nightingales: The Emergence of the Nursing Profession at Bellevue and New York Hospital, 1850–1920.* Ann Arbor, Mich.: UMI Research Press, 1981.

Mulvany, Esther Ring. *Lamps Still Aglow: A History of Kansas Nursing.* North Newton, Kans.: Mennonite Press, 1976.

National League of Nursing Education. *Proceedings of Annual Conventions,* 1912–1950.

Nellie Nelson, "Image of Nursing: Influences of the Present." In *Nursing Today: Transition and Trends,* edited by JoAnn Zerwekh and Jo Carol Claborn, 53–83. Philadelphia: Saunders, 2000.

Nelson, Sioban. "Entering the Professional Domain: The Making of the Modern Nurse in 17th Century France." *Nursing History Review* 7 (1999): 171–87.

———. *Say Little, Do Much: Nurses, Nuns, and Hospitals in the Nineteenth Century.* Philadelphia: University of Pennsylvania Press, 2001.

Newman, Margaret. "Toward an Integrative Model of Professional Practice." *Journal of Professional Nursing* 6 (May–June 1990): 167–73.

Newman, Margaret A., A. Marilyn Sime, and Sheila A. Corcoran-Perry. "The Focus of the Discipline of Nursing." *Advances in Nursing Science* 14 (September 1991): 1–6.

"New Party Is Forming; May Invade State." *St. Paul Pioneer Press,* July 1, 1918, 1.

Nightingale, Florence. Letter to Mary Jones (Superintendent of St. John's nurses at University College Hospital, 1867). In *As Miss Nightingale Said . . . ,* edited by Monica Baly, 96. London: Scutari Press, 1991.

———. *Notes on Nursing: What It Is and What It Is Not.* 2d ed. Norwalk, Conn.: Appleton-Century-Crofts, 1860; reprint, New York: Dover Publications, 1969.

———. "Sick Nursing and Health Nursing." In *Hospitals, Dispensaries, and Nursing, International Congress of Charities, Correction, and Philanthropy, Sec. III, Held in Chicago June 15–17, 1893,* edited by J. S. Billings and H. M. Hurd, 444–63. Baltimore: Johns Hopkins Press, 1894.

Noddings, Nel. *Caring: A Feminine Approach to Ethics and Moral Education.* Berkeley: University of California Press, 1984.

Norman, Linda. "Continuous Improvement in Nursing Education." *IHI Quality Connection* 6 (spring 1997): 4.

"Northwest Conditions Termed Satisfactory." *St. Paul Pioneer Press,* October 6, 1929, 1.

"Nurse Membership in Unions." *American Journal of Nursing* 37 (July 1937): 766–67.

Nutting, Mary Adelaide. *A Sound Economic Basis for Schools of Nursing and Other Addresses.* New York: G. P. Putnam's, 1926.

Nutting, Mary Adelaide. "The Outlook in Nursing." In *Proceedings of the Twenty-Sixth Annual Convention of the National League of Nursing Education,* 309–10. Baltimore: Williams and Wilkins, 1921.

Oderkirk, Wendell W. "'Organize or Perish': The Transformation of Nebraska Nursing Education, 1888–1941." Ph.D. diss., University of Nebraska, 1988.

———. "A Peculiar and Valuable Service." *Nebraska History* 80 (summer 1999): 66–79.

———. "Setting the Record Straight: A Recount of Late Nineteenth-Century Training Schools." *Journal of Nursing History* 1 (November 1985): 30–37.

Olson, Thomas C. "The Women of St. Luke's and the Evolution of Nursing, 1892–1937." Ph.D. diss., University of Minnesota, 1991.

Olson, Tom. "Apprenticeship and Exploitation: An Analysis of the Work Pattern of Nurses in Training, 1897–1937." *Social Science History* 17 (winter 1993): 559–76.

———. "Balancing Theory and Practice in Nursing Education: Case Study of a Historic Struggle." *Nursing Outlook* 46 (November/December 1998): 268–72.

———. "Competing Paradigms and the St. Luke's Alumnae Association Minutes, 1895–1916." *Advances in Nursing Science* 12 (June 1990): 53–62.

———. "Laying Claim to Caring: Nursing and the Language of Training." *Nursing Outlook* 41 (March–April 1993): 68–72.

———. "Numbers, Narratives, and Nursing History." *Social Science Journal* 37 (January 2000): 137–44.

———. "Recreating Past Separations and the Employment Pattern of Nurses." *Nursing Outlook,* 43 (September/October 1995): 210–14.

———. "The Women of St. Luke's and the Occupational Evolution of Nursing, 1897–1915." *Mid-America, An Historical Review* 73 (April–July 1991): 109–26.

Osler, William. *Nurse and Patient.* Baltimore: John Murphy and Company, 1897.

Partridge, Rebecca. "Education for Entry into Professional Nursing Practice: The Planning of Change." *Journal of Nursing Education* 20 (April 1981): 40–46.

Passau-Buck, Shirlee. "Caring vs. Curing: The Politics of Health Care." In *Socialization, Sexism, and Stereotyping,* edited by Janet Muff, 203–209. Prospect Heights, Ill.: Waveland Press, 1982.

Pence, Terry, and Janice Cantrall. "Philosophical Foundations of Nursing Practice." In *Ethics in Nursing: An Anthology,* edited by Terry Pence and Janice Cantrall, 1–9. New York: National League for Nursing, 1990.

Pope, William C. *The Church in St. Paul.* St Paul: Minnesota Historical Society, 1911.

Porter, Sam. "The Poverty of Professionalization: A Critical Analysis of Strategies for the Occupational Advancement of Nursing." *Journal of Advanced Nursing* 17 (June 1992): 720–26.

Powell, David. "Nurses—Sacrificial Lambs of Healthcare." *RN* 64 (January 2001): 51–52.

Procedures Used in the Teaching of the Principles and Practice of Nursing. St. Paul: Children's Hospital, 1930.

"Protection of Girls Planned in Capital." *St. Paul Pioneer Press,* July 7, 1918, 10.

Rachleff, Peter. "Turning Points in the Labor Movement: Three Key Conflicts." In *Minnesota in a Century of Change: The State and Its People Since 1900,* edited by Clifford E. Clark Jr., 195–222. St. Paul: Minnesota Historical Society, 1989.

Rajabally, M. H. "Point of View: The Entry into Practice Issue, We Have Seen the Enemy." *Canadian Nurse* 78 (February 1982): 40, 42.

Ramos, Mary Carol. "The Johns Hopkins Training School for Nurses: A Tale of Vision, Labor, and Futility." *Nursing History Review* 5 (1997): 23–48

Rankiellour, Caroline M. "The Minnesota State Registered Association." *Minnesota Registered Nurse* 3 (October 1930): 13–19.

Ream, Alice. "Our Undertrained Nurses." *Newsweek* 100, October 21, 1982, 17.

Reed, Pamela G. "Nursing Reformation: Historical Reflections and Philosophic Foundations." *Nursing Science Quarterly* 13 (April 2000): 129–36.

Reeves, M. Sandra, and Warren Cohen. "College Guide." *U.S. News and World Report,* October 15, 1990, 124.

Reskin, Barbara F. "Bringing the Men Back In: Sex Differentiation and the Devaluation of Women's Work." *Gender and Society* 2 (March 1988): 58–81.

Reverby, Susan M. "'Neither for the Drawing Room nor for the Kitchen': Private Duty Nursing in Boston, 1873–1920." In *Women and Health in America: Historical Readings,* edited by Judith Walzer Leavitt, 454–66. Madison: University of Wisconsin Press, 1984.

———. *Ordered to Care: The Dilemma of American Nursing, 1850–1945.* Cambridge: Cambridge University Press, 1987.

———. "The Search for the Hospital Yardstick: Nursing and the Rationalization of Hospital Work." In *Sickness and Health in America: Readings in the History of Medicine and Public Health,* 2d ed., edited by Judith Walzer Leavitt and Ronald L. Numbers, 206–16. Madison: University of Wisconsin Press, 1985.

Riley, Glenda. "In or Out of the Historical Kitchen." *Minnesota History* 52 (summer 1990): 61–71.

Robb, Isabel Hampton. *Educational Standards for Nurses with Other Addresses on Nursing Subjects.* Cleveland: E. C. Koeckert, 1905/1907.

Roberts, Mary M. *American Nursing: History and Interpretation.* New York: Macmillan, 1954.

Rogers, Naomi. *An Alternative Path: The Making and Remaking of Hahnemann Medical College and Hospital of Philadelphia.* Rutgers: Rutgers University Press, 1998.

Rorabaugh, W. J. *The Craft Apprentice: From Franklin to the Machine Age in America.* New York: Oxford University Press, 1986.

Rosenberg, Charles E. *The Care of Strangers.* Cambridge, England: Cambridge University Press, 1987.

Rosener, J. "Ways Women Lead." *Harvard Business Review* 68 (1990): 119–25.

Ross, Jack C. *An Assembly of Good Fellows: Voluntary Associations in History.* Westport, Conn.: Greenwood Press, 1976.

Ruggles, Steven. *Prolonged Connections: The Rise of the Extended Family in Nineteenth-Century England and America.* Madison: University of Wisconsin Press, 1987.

"St. Paul Women Rally to Call for Great Increase in Knitting." *St. Paul Pioneer Press,* July 7, 1918, 4.

Salvage, J. *The Politics of Nursing.* London: Heinemann, 1985.

Sandelowki, Margarete. *Devices and Desires: Gender, Technology, and American Nursing.* Chapel Hill, N.C.: University of North Carolina Press, 2000.

Sassler, Sharon, and Michael J. White. "Ethnicity, Gender, and Social Mobility in 1910." *Social Science History* 21 (fall 1997): 321–49.

Schroedel, Jean Reith. *Alone in a Crowd: Women in the Trades Tell Their Stories.* Philadelphia: Temple University Press, 1985.

Schwirian, Patricia M. *Professionalization of Nursing: Current Issues and Trends.* Philadelphia: Lippincott, 1998.

Scott, Joan Wallach. *Gender and the Politics of History.* New York: Columbia University Press, 1988.

———. "Gender: A Useful Category of Historical Analysis." *American Historical Review* 91 (December 1986): 1053–75.

Selanders, Louise C. "Florence Nightingale: The Evolution and Social Impact of Feminist Values in Nursing." *Journal of Holistic Nursing* 16 (June 1998): 247–63.

Shryock, Henry S., and Jacob S. Siegel. *The Methods and Materials of Demography.* Washington, D.C.: Department of Commerce, Bureau of the Census, 1980.

Smith, Marlaine C. "The Distinctiveness of Nursing Knowledge." *Nursing Science Quarterly* 5 (winter 1992): 148–49.

Smith, Susan L. *Sick and Tired of Being Sick and Tired: Black Women's Health Activism in America, 1890–1950.* Philadelphia: University of Pennsylvania Press, 1995.

Smola, Bonnie Ketchum. "A Study of the Development of Diploma and Baccalaureate Degree Nursing Education Programs in Iowa from 1907–1978." Ph.D. diss., Iowa State University, 1980.

Smuts, Robert. *Women and Work in America.* New York: Columbia University Press, 1959.

Sobek, Mathew. "Class Analysis and the U.S. Census Public Use Samples." *Historical Methods* 24 (fall 1991): 171–82.

Starr, Paul. *The Social Transformation of Medicine.* New York: Basic Books, 1982.

Steinberg, Ronnie J. "Gendered Instructions: Cultural Lag and Gender Bias in the Hay System of Job Evaluation." *Work and Occupations* 19 (November 1992): 387–423.

———. "Social Construction of Skill: Gender, Power, and Comparable Worth." *Work and Occupations* 17 (November 1990): 449–82.

Stewart, Isabel. "The Science and Art of Nursing, Editorial." *Nursing Education Bulletin* 2 (1929): 1.

Stewart, Isabel Maitland. *The Education of Nurses: Historical Foundations and Modern Trends.* New York: Macmillan, 1944.

Stewart, Isabel Maitland, and Anne S. Austin. *A History of Nursing from Ancient to Modern Times—A World View.* 5th ed. New York: G. P. Putnam's Sons, 1962.

Stivers, C. *Gender Images in Public Administration.* London: Sage, 1993.

Strachan, Glenda. *Labour of Love: The History of the Nurses' Association in Queensland, 1860–1950.* Sydney: Allen and Unwin, 1996.

Styles, Margaretta, Sheila Allen, Sara Armstrong, Marsha Matsura, Daphne Stannard, and Julia Stocker Ordway. "Entry: A New Approach." *Nursing Outlook* 39 (September–October 1991): 200–3.

Swanson, Kristen M. "Empirical Development of a Middle Range Theory of Caring." *Nursing Research* 40 (May/June 1991): 161–66.

Swift, Fletcher Harper. "The Increasing Professionalization of Educational Workers." In *Changing Educational World,* edited by Alvin C. Eurich, 205. Minneapolis: University of Minnesota Press, 1931.

Tannen, D. *You Just Don't Understand: Women and Men in Conversation.* London: Virago, 1991.

Tanner, Rev. George C. *Fifty Years of Church Work in the Diocese of Minnesota, 1857–1907.* St. Paul: The Committee, 1909.

"Temperance Rally: Twin City Good Templars Hold a Joint Meeting." *St. Paul Pioneer Press,* March 2, 1897, 3.

Tenth Anniversary of the Swedish Hospital, 1898–1908. Minneapolis: Swedish Hospital, 1908 (on permanent deposit with the Minnesota Historical Society).

Tentler, Leslie Woodcock. *Wage-Earning Women: Industrial Work and Family Life in the United States, 1900–1930.* New York: Oxford University Press, 1979.

Thayer, Steve. *Saint Mudd.* Washington, D.C.: Pilot Grove Press, 1988.

Tilly, Louise A., and Joan W. Scott. *Women, Work, and Family.* New York: Holt, Rinehart and Winston, 1978.

Titus, Shirley C., and Margaret Huey. "Appointment to the Faculty." *American Journal of Nursing* 36 (June 1936): 597–601.

"To Bob or Not to Bob." *St. Paul Pioneer Press,* October 1, 1924, 1.

"To Stop Smoking among Our Youths." *St. Paul Pioneer Press,* July 1, 1900, 24.

Tomes, Nancy. "The Silent Battle: Nurse Registration in New York State, 1903–1920." In *Nursing History: New Perspectives, New Possibilities,* edited by Ellen Condliffe Lagemann, 107–32. New York: Teachers College Press, 1983.

————. "'Little World of Our Own': The Pennsylvania Hospital Training School for Nurses, 1895–1907." In *Women and Health in America: Historical Readings,* edited by Judith Walzer Leavitt, 467–81. Madison: University of Wisconsin Press, 1984.

Trachtenberg, Alan. *The Incorporation of America: Culture and Society in the Gilded Age.* New York: Hill and Wang, 1982.

Treiman, Donald J., and Heidi Hartmann, eds. *Women, Work and Wages: Equal Pay for Jobs of Equal Value.* Washington, D.C.: National Academy Press, 1981.

Tschirch, Poldi, ed. *A Century of Excellence, A Vision for the Future: The University of Texas School of Nursing at Galveston, 1890–1990.* Galveston: University of Texas Medical Branch, 1990.

"The Twin Cities Are Lousy." *Milwaukee Journal,* September 14, 1933, 4.

"Union Membership? No!" *American Journal of Nursing* 38 (May 1938): 573–74.

"U.S. Airmen Victors in Fierce Half-hour Fight." *St. Paul Pioneer Press,* July 3, 1918, 1.

von Conrad, Georgia Bernadette. "The First Eighty Years: The History of Lutheran Medical Center School of Nursing, 1898–1978." Ph.D. diss., Saint Louis University, 1980.

Waerness, K. "On the Rationality of Caring." In *Women and the State,* edited by A. Showstack Sassoon. London: Routledge, 1984.

"Wage Purity War on Wickedness." *St. Paul Pioneer Press,* October 1, 1910, 12.

Walsh, Eileen. *The Last Resort: Northern Minnesota Tourism and the Integration of Rural and Urban Worlds, 1900–1950.* Ph.D. diss., University of Minnesota, 1994.

Wandersee, Winifred D. *Women's Work and Family Values, 1920–1940.* Cambridge, Mass.: Harvard University Press, 1981.

Watkins, Carolyn. "The Redefinition of Professional Nursing: The Aultman Hospital School of Nursing Experience." Ph.D. diss., University of Akron, 1987.

Watson, Jean. *Nursing: Human Science and Human Care.* Norwalk, Conn.: Appleton-Century-Crofts, 1988.

————. *Nursing: The Philosophy and Science of Caring.* Boulder: Colorado Associated University Press, 1985.

Watson, Jean, and Sally Phillips. "A Call for Educational Reform: Colorado Nursing Doctorate Model as Exemplar." *Nursing Outlook* 40 (1992): 20–26.

Weiner, Lynn. "Our Sister's Keeper": The Minneapolis Women's Christian Association and Housing for Working Women." *Minnesota History* 46 (spring 1979): 189–200.

"What Will You Do?" *Trained Nurse and Hospital Review* 107 (November 1941): 367.

"Why Join?" *American Journal of Nursing* 36 (October 1930): 1021–22.

Wilder, Laura Ingalls. *By the Shores of Silver Lake.* New York: Harper and Row, 1953.

———. *On the Banks of Plum Creek.* New York: Harper and Row, 1953.

Wilensky, Harold L. "The Professionalization of Everyone?" *American Journal of Sociology* 70 (1964): 137–58.

William-Evans, Shiprah A. Alicia, and M. Elizabeth Carnegie. "The Evolution of Professional Nursing." In *Contemporary Nursing: Issues, Trends, and Management,* edited by Barbara Cherry and Susan R. Jacob, 1–25. St. Louis, Mo.: Mosby, 2002.

Wilson, Leonard. *Medical Revolution in Minnesota: A History of the University of Minnesota Medical School.* St. Paul: Midewiwin Press, 1989.

Wolf, Karen Anne, ed. *Jo Ann Ashley: Selected Readings.* New York: NLN Press, 1997.

Wolf, Margaret S. "Group Stages: One View of the Development of the Nursing Profession." *Image* 9 (October 1977): 64–67.

Woods, Cynthia Q. "From Individual Dedication to Social Activism: Historical Development of Nursing Professionalism." In *Nursing History: The State of the Art,* edited by Christopher Maggs, 153–75. Wolfeboro, N.H.: Croom Helm, 1987.

Index

20–21, 27, 31–38, 44–46, 54–57, 72

medicine v. nursing, 11, 14–15, 84–86, 153, 185n. 36
Melosh, 5, 49, 64, 115, 153
Minnesota: early-twentieth-century development, 25–28; during World War I, 59–60; epidemics, 104–5; fire, 105; nursing collective action organizations, 128–29
models of nursing, 1–8, 14, 31–38, 52–53, 60–68, 91–94, 129, 132–33, 142, 145–55, 157n. 4, 158n. 9, 204n. 52. *See also* professionalization framework

Nightingale, Florence, 2–3, 14–15, 37, 44, 86, 129, 144, 153
nurses' registry, St. Paul, 16, 72–73, 128–32, 137
nursing: anti-intellectualism, 32; definitions of, 82, 92–94 (*see* models of nursing); elite, 1, 4, 32, 53, 93, 130, 132, 143, 145–48, 151–52; friendships, 136–38; and higher education, 31–32, 94–95, 114–15, 133, 143–44; job mobility, 135–37, 139–40; labor organizing, 65–68, 106–9, 122–26, 128–30; lesbians, 11; male exclusion, 14–15; marital status, 16–18, 46, 109–11, 124, 138–39; moral emphasis, 14, 44–45, 57,118–20; need for, 11; personality traits, 112–14; and practicality, 2–3, 31, 57, 107–9, 123, 127–29, 168n. 114; private duty, 16, 37, 65, 70, 95, 125–26, 137, 144–46; professionalization of, 2–4, 25, 30–32, 93, 123, 132, 145, 148–55 (*see* professionalization framework); public service aspect, 39–49, 122–23; rank-and-file nurses, 4, 6–7, 67, 84, 92, 115, 129, 155; as religious calling, 40–44; salary, 133–35, 144; and social movements, 131; women's unique ability for, 14, 19, 40,

44–46, 48–49, 86, 93 (*see* gender); work, on duty, 60–72, 78–94, 133
Nutting, Adelaide, 30, 53, 62, 95, 182n. 75

occupational opportunities for women, 27–29, 32–38, 114, 121–22; school teaching, 32, 36–37,141

physical strength, stature and endurance, 21–24, 37–38, 57, 92 94, 103–7, 120, 149–50
professionalization framework, 1, 3–5, 93, 123, 127–33, 140–42, 145–46, 154. *See also* models of nursing

Ramsey County Graduate Nurses' Association (aka Nurses' Association), 15–16, 128, 131
religion and nursing, 3, 38, 40–44, 150
Reverby, 26, 44–45, 123

St. Luke's Hospital and Training School for Nurses: application information, 7–8; 13–23, 25–26, 29–38, 42, 45–52; Alumnae Association, 122–23; Board of Managers (female), 12; Board of Physicians (male), 13; Board of Trustees (male), 12, 43; daily life, 59–60, 83, 101; dismissals of nurse trainees, 96–99, 117–20; instructions to entering nurses, 1, 9; lady managers 12–13; legacy, 146, 149, 152–54; male exclusion, 15; moral requirements, 45–46, 108–10, 113–14, 116–20, 195n. 141; physical setting, 9, 13, 29; religious aspects, 40–44, 59; reputation of school, 28, 48, 130, 143; resignations of nurse trainees, 99–120; rural backgrounds, 25–26, 29; standards for admission, 30; pay (stipend), 28, 52, 95; training program decreased, 60; Training

Reproductive Health, Reproductive Rights: Reformers and the Politics of Maternal Welfare, 1917–1940
Robyn L. Rosen

Women and Prenatal Testing: Facing the Challenges of Genetic Technology
Edited by Karen H. Rothenberg and Elizabeth J. Thomson

Women's Health: Complexities and Differences
Edited by Sheryl Burt Ruzek, Virginia L. Olesen, and Adele E. Clarke

Bodies of Technology: Women's Involvement with Reproductive Medicine
Edited by Ann R. Saetnan, Nelly Oudshoorn, and Marty Kirejczyk

Motherhood in Bondage
Margaret Sanger. Foreword by Margaret Marsh

Listen to Me Good: The Life Story of an Alabama Midwife
Margaret Charles Smith and Linda Janet Holmes

Don't Kill Your Baby: Public Health and the Decline of Breastfeeding in the Nineteenth and Twentieth Centuries
Jacqueline H. Wolf